CHRONIC DISEASE AND DISABILITY

A Basic Medical-Social Guide

CHRONIC
and

DISEASE
DISABILITY

by GEORGIA TRAVIS

UNIVERSITY OF CALIFORNIA PRESS 1961
Berkeley and Los Angeles

UNIVERSITY OF CALIFORNIA PRESS
BERKELEY AND LOS ANGELES, CALIFORNIA
CAMBRIDGE UNIVERSITY PRESS
LONDON, ENGLAND
© 1961 BY THE REGENTS OF THE UNIVERSITY OF CALIFORNIA
LIBRARY OF CONGRESS CATALOG NUMBER: 61–7519
PRINTED IN THE UNITED STATES OF AMERICA

Foreword

Increased availability of federal and state funds for medical care has given the caseworker long desired invaluable means for more nearly total care of the needy.

Correlation of the effects of an illness with the recipient's social, mental and financial state is too frequently hampered by incomplete knowledge and lack of information concerning the illness in question. Because of the current availability of more complete medical data about given recipients, caseworkers must have an amplified working knowledge of certain diseases and their possible and probable social effects on the patient and his associates.

This volume is designed to give social workers a central focal point from which to obtain technical medical information combined with empirical knowledge of resulting social effects.

Georgia Travis ably presents some of the most prevalent

chronic illnesses in capsule fashion, selecting the medical facts that have social consequences or would be of special interest to social workers. She has used accepted medical sources and gives authenticated information. The strength and purpose of her book are augmented by her sound comments on the social impact of the various diseases upon the patient and his family.

JOHN D. KEYE, M.D.

Preface

Illness and disability are common in public assistance case-loads, both because prolonged illness creates poverty and because the underprivileged are especially liable to disabling illness. When an infection occurs that would be transitory in an individual with high resistance, it is likely to become entrenched in the poor man's system.

The poor man tends to postpone medical care because of its cost or because of the inconvenience of clinic care; when he has a long-time illness such as diabetes or heart disease, he may develop disabling complications because of the lack of proper food, medicine, warmth, and rest.

No item in the client's life is more important than his health. Freedom from pain, apathy, and physical restriction is essential to vigorous pursuit of employment and to concentrated consideration of how to better one's lot.

Constructive social planning requires a knowledge of the client's medical condition. Is his illness fatal? Is it infectious? Is it repulsive? How long will it incapacitate him? Is it painful, debilitating? Should we budget for increased diet, carfare, fuel, extra night clothes, sturdy shoes, a heating pad?

Are the treatments something anyone would try to avoid? Is the illness one that would frighten any family? Will it separate the client from his family? Will it change his accustomed role? Our knowledge of the social and emotional repercussions caused by the illness is prerequisite to our understanding and our planning.

What of the badly disabled person, or the frail elderly client known to have a long-time disease? His condition may shift and vary, getting worse for lack of material things, worry, or enough supervision; or it may get better under some treatment he is having, so that he can be considered in a different light than when he applied for assistance.

Long-time conditions are neither static nor hopeless; much can be done to reduce further disability or discomfort, and often what can be done medically is made possible by social means. Money for a drug sometimes prevents a stroke, a properly placed pillow may prevent deformity, help with a diet may prevent hospitalization or even save a life. What dramatic results accrue from prosaic ways!

These things are obvious. Yet social workers in all kinds of agencies frequently slide over health matters. We tend to feel helpless about illness, to think it is all the doctor's affair, or to think that everything is "emotional."

Possibly one explanation is that it is difficult to secure information from doctors or hospitals. Perhaps the most important reason for this is lack of sufficient knowledge to know what to ask, or to understand such technical information as is obtained. Medical terminology is complex and seems shrouded in mystery; even a doctor's handwriting may be difficult to read, let alone the substance of what he has written down.

The purpose of the book is to provide a summary of socially pertinent medical facts about common chronic diseases of adults, which can be used as a starting point in securing needed information. The practical meaning of these diseases is described with recognition that a wide range of variation occurs depending upon the client and his social situation as well as upon the severity of the disease.

The social implications emphasized in this book are those that relate to matters of budget, environmental service, counseling, and work with other agencies and professions. In other words, this book is slanted to the physical reality of the sick or disabled client and to the tangible services which can help make his medical care effective and help him be more comfortable.

Each chapter has been written to stand by itself, so that the worker who is in a hurry can read the book a chapter at a time, choosing the chapter that may be most helpful at the time. The social implications of various chronic diseases are closely allied. In an effort not to repeat extensively, certain topics are elaborated in one chapter and not in another. It is assumed that the worker will soon have read most of the chapters and will carry over from one part to the other; also that by using the index she can find a discussion in which she is especially interested at a certain time.

The book was begun as a training aid to be used in conjunction with the Aid to Disabled program of the California State Department of Social Welfare, after a search had failed to reveal any book providing a simple explanation of chronic disease and disability with their social implications. The many pamphlets issued by certain organizations regarding disease entities that concern them are, of course, of great value, as are the periodical articles about the social and emotional implications of various diseases, but a more comprehensive statement seemed a practical need.

Superficially, it may seem that medical information should be presented by a physician, and public assistance information by a public assistance specialist. But it is the relationship between the medical and social situations, or the practical implications of the illness, which has received emphasis here. This bridge between medicine and social work has been literally named "medical-social" work.

Notable omissions occur in the book. The largest has to do with children's diseases. These were not included because my affiliation has been with a program which serves only adults. Especially regretted are omissions of alcoholism and suicide. The physical and mental consequences of alcoholism have become major medical-social problems, as is well known. Suicide, the seventh leading cause of death, also merits discussion in a book for social workers about chronic disease, because concern over ill health is a major cause of the suicides which could have been prevented if there had been someone to listen and care. Unfortunately, lack of time for a comprehensive compilation prevented the inclusion of chapters on these conditions.

The information in the book incorporates technical terms commonly used. Most of these are not only listed in a glossary at the end of each chapter, but are used in the narrative. Those not found in the glossary are explained in the text. The purpose is to acquaint the worker with the terms she will hear the physician use and that she will see in medical reports.

The medical information presented here is taken from a variety of sources which are listed in the bibliography. All medical statements have been edited by physicians.

The social implications and suggestions represent my own views. Their applicability to public assistance has been checked by experts and practitioners in the California state and local welfare departments, but they do not necessarily represent the policies of these departments.

Acknowledgments

This volume, though by no means an official document, is a product of the California State Department of Social Welfare. Mr. Leon Lefson, Chief of the Bureau of Aid to the Needy Disabled, and Mrs. Elizabeth B. MacLatchie, Chief of the Division of Social Security, encouraged the idea of the book and provided me with an opportunity to write it.

Mr. J. M. Wedemeyer, Director of the Department of Social Welfare, has fostered efforts of the staff toward increased understanding of the needs of people and of ways to help.

A book which incorporates medical information could not be written by a lay person without the generous help of physicians. John D. Keye, M.D., Medical Director of the Department of Social Welfare, did most of the medical editing, with the assistance of L. E. McDonald, M.D., Sacramento Area Medical Consultant, and John D. Keye, Jr., M.D. Frank Cline, Jr., M.D., Tuberculosis Control Officer, Sacramento County Department of Public Health, edited the chapter on tuberculosis; William Ball, M.D., cardiologist, edited the chapter on cardiovascular disease. Herbert Bauer, M.D., Health Officer, Yolo County, California, Department of Public Health, read the entire manuscript.

I am deeply indebted to these physicians, not only for their time and patience in evaluating the accuracy of simplified medical information, but for their helpful comments and suggestions.

Various members of the staff of the State Department of Social Welfare, including Mrs. Rebecca Gentile and Miss Grace Nichols, read parts of the manuscript and gave much-appreciated criticism. Mrs. Agnes Gregory, Public Assistance Specialist in the Bureau of Old Age Security, used her great store of knowledge of public assistance to determine the feasibility of suggestions made in the sections called "Implications for Public Assistance."

Mrs. Dilla Ludlow cheerfully rendered invaluable assistance in finding reference materials. Mrs. Jo Capps and Miss Laura Shiroi first typed the difficult manuscript; Mrs. Dorothy Flanigan and her staff commented helpfully on the content as well as engaging in the long, exacting task of typing the final draft.

A number of staff members from Humboldt, Santa Clara, Riverside, and Sacramento county departments of public welfare, and individual staff members from many other county departments helped pretest parts of the manuscript. I am especially indebted to them for their time and interest and their response and suggestions.

Several other persons and organizations helped significantly. The California Tuberculosis Association compiled the glossary for the chapter on tuberculosis, with staff work by Mrs. Trude Baum. Mr. Arpad Kertesz of the Sacramento Alcoholic Rehabilitation Clinic and Mr. James Boock, Chief of General Assistance—Aid to Disabled Division, Sacramento County Department of Public Welfare, shared their experience in the treatment of the tuberculous alcoholic.

The following persons generously provided information

and literature on the subjects of their special concern: Mrs. Claya Budd, Executive Director of the Arthritis and Rheumatism Foundation, San Francisco; Mrs. Majorie Brush, Executive Director, United Cerebral Palsy Association, San Francisco; and Mrs. Thelma Dawson of the Sacramento Chapter of the American Cancer Society.

Permission to quote from comments made by Blanche D. Gubersky, R.N., in *The Care of the Geriatric Patient* was kindly given by E. V. Cowdry, the editor, and by the publisher, the C. V. Mosby Company. Sincere thanks are expressed to them, and to Dan Morse, M.D., who gave permission to quote from his article, "Alcohol and Tuberculosis," published in the National Tuberculosis Association *Bulletin* in November, 1956.

G. T.

Contents

CHAPTER I

Working with the Chronically Ill

WORKING WITH THE CHRONICALLY ILL and disabled is interesting and often rewarding. It is a coöperative venture. This eases the task, but it also adds complexity. Being one of a group means that the worker can depend upon others to carry out the responsibilities for which they are equipped and she is not.* However, it also means that she is expected to make her own unique contribution, to relate this contribution to the efforts of the others, and, above all, to make sure that the client or recipient gets the benefit of the services of the whole group and does not fall between.

In other words, the public welfare worker need not be held back from services to the chronically ill by fear of involving herself in activities that are beyond her scope. Physician and nurse will supply physical care and advice. Medical social workers in hospitals or health agencies, voca-

---

* For convenience, the worker will be referred to as "she" and the client, or recipient, as "he," throughout the book.

tional rehabilitation counselors, clergymen, dietitians, physical and occupational therapists—all will be available in various numbers and combinations, depending upon the community and the recipient's situation, to provide their skills as needed.

The public welfare worker's own specific responsibilities or the contribution she makes to the total group effort in behalf of the recipient are: to determine eligibility for public assistance; to decide on the appropriate categorical aid; to compute the budget; to make critical decisions involving agency funds and community resources, such as those relating to out-of-home care; to counsel with the client and family about matters that will be affected by the client's health; to help the client secure medical care if he needs it; to use the resources of the agency and community in assisting the client in using medical care effectively.

It can readily be seen that each one of these is a legitimate and a familiar function. On close examination it becomes clear, however, that none of these duties can be performed adequately in behalf of the chronically ill or disabled person unless the worker understands the illness and its social implications.

This book describes the general ways in which the illness affects the client and the worker's planning. The worker will need to rely on the client's physician for specific information about how the illness affects the particular client, and upon the client and his family for an understanding of what the disability means to him.

In addition to carrying on her own appropriate functions, the social worker often finds herself the liaison person, the coördinator, the catalyst, the interpreter. She often initiates services from others and then follows through to be certain of the client's understanding and acceptance of recommendations and of his ability to carry them out.

The worker may have no question about her responsibilities, but feel hampered in working with chronically ill clients by a sense of uneasiness in being around sick people. Many social workers, in common with the rest of humanity, have some uncomfortable feelings about illness. If a worker finds that this feeling does not diminish and she is having continued reluctance to visit sick or disabled clients, it is well to search for the reasons and to talk the matter over with the supervisor. An eminent social worker of my acquaintance cannot be around sick people at all. This does happen occasionally, and is no disgrace. Caseloads sometimes have to be transferred, or individual cases shifted to other workers, because of the very real barriers which a worker's feelings can create. Fortunately most workers eventually become comfortable in working with the sick or disabled and, in fact, find it an opportunity for challenging and satisfying service.

The Client and His Family

THE INTERVIEW

Interviewing a sick person requires the same principles of courtesy and common sense that underlie interviewing the well, and which would obtain in calling on a sick friend. The major problems in conducting the interview are to avoid staying too long or disturbing the person when unpleasant facts have to be discussed. Checking with the physician or the caretaker in advance of any particularly difficult discussions (such as budget cuts, overpayments, out-of-home care) may be indicated if the person has a condition in which nervous strain may be physically harmful, such as diabetes, thyroid disease, heart disease, high blood pressure, colitis, or rheumatoid arthritis.

How much should the worker burden the client with, and how much should be discussed with the spouse, adult child, or caretaker? One determinant is the usual or pre-illness role of the person in the family. A mother will still expect to make decisions about or discuss the problems of her child; a father (in most instances), matters of budget and family moves; the individual, his own hospital placement or change in living plans. On the other hand, a person who has been sick a long time and has turned over the management of his affairs, let us say, to an adult child, will usually welcome freedom from having to think about budget details, verification of special needs, or worrisome detailed plans for the future.

The fact that the person is in a supine position or sitting in a wheel chair does not disqualify him from participating in an interview. The sick person should be addressed directly and by name. A natural tendency seems to exist to exclude the sick person and to refer to him as "he," as if being ill made him deaf and dumb. It is how much participation to invite, not the fact of participation, which requires judgment. This judgment is based not only on the former role of the person and the content of the discussion but primarily by how acutely or seriously ill he is. Many disabling conditions are relatively static; for example, a crippled person may not be sick to the extent of being in actual distress. In an interview the person who is crippled from poliomyelitis or the early multiple-sclerosis victim is a vastly different person from a suffering arthritic or an enfeebled cancer patient. A person who is acutely ill, with a high temperature or in severe pain, or who is seriously ill and debilitated should not be interviewed at all.

"The client is the best source of information," a basic premise in interviewing the well, does not apply to the sick person so far as his medical condition is concerned.

The sick client often has a distorted or incomplete picture, either because the doctor did not give him a complete story or because he blocked out what he heard or misunderstood what the physician wished to convey. So that the worker will understand the actual medical problem, she should ask the client if he has any objection to her talking with his doctor. If he has none, the physician should be approached for information.

The client (and the person responsible for his care) is, however, the best source of information about what the disability means to him from a practical standpoint. This information is secondary in importance only to a knowledge of the medical condition as obtained from the doctor. The best way to find out what a disability means to an individual is to get him to talk about his condition—that is, how long he has been disabled, the cause, his symptoms, the treatment he has had, and what life has been like for him since. Drawing out a person about what he can and cannot do often requires gentle interrogation, because ill persons get so accustomed to their routines that they find them difficult to describe. A common device is having the client describe a usual day or what he did yesterday.

Most persons like to talk about themselves and their illness, and welcome a listener who is interested in details. As in any interviewing, the worker's responsibility is to guide the interview rather than merely to sit and listen to whatever happens to be on the client's mind at the moment. Therefore, there is no reason why the worker should not guide the interview in such a way that she gets a clear understanding of how the disability or illness interferes with the client's former way of functioning or the disappointment and frustration it has meant to him.

If the worker observes that the client is becoming too upset or anxious or that the conversation is becoming distressing to him, she will stop probing, give the client a chance to collect himself, and tactfully pick up on a brighter aspect of his situation. No hard-and-fast rules exist. The worker must use sensitivity and judgment in this, as in everything else. The point is that she need not avoid the whole issue of how a disability has affected the client's life. Far from it—we must know, and the client needs and often enjoys an opportunity to talk about it.

An ironclad rule is that no one but a physician may reveal knowledge of the individual's physical condition to him. This is an old, well-established principle of ethics which must never be violated. How does the worker learn what the client knows or thinks about his condition? "What did the doctor say the last time he was here?" or "What does the doctor say about your condition?" is the kind of question a worker may use to discover what the client thinks about his condition or how much he understands. By listening, nodding, commenting briefly—in other words, by the usual interviewing technique—the worker can determine the areas she can safely explore.

If the worker learns that the client has a different understanding of his illness than the doctor has conveyed to the worker, and if there is no reason to feel that the doctor would deliberately withhold information on the subject, the worker should arrange for the client to talk with the doctor again. It is necessary to let the doctor know in advance about the client's apparent misunderstanding and to ask that the doctor discuss the medical situation again with the client. The worker should tell the doctor why she is asking that this be done—for example, either that the patient's peace of mind has been jeopardized by misunderstanding or that some practical matter such as employment, schooling, diet, activity limitation, or family problem is affected by the client's lack of understanding of the implications of his medical condition.

THE SICK OR DISABLED PERSON

Illness is not usually an abrupt change in state of being, but a point gradually reached and gradually receded from. All kinds of variations exist along the continuum from the rather academic state of "normal health" to "disease." Feeling unwell, the sick person is not free to concentrate upon things outside himself but is preoccupied with his distress. He fatigues quickly; he is in a vulnerable position; he requires the help of the well.

Psychology is so intertwined with physiology that the person who is physically dependent is also psychologically dependent. Not only does he need to lean physically, but he feels a need to lean emotionally. Feeling a need for dependence is a complicated matter for adults because it evokes the childhood situation, which may not have been ideal. A short bout of dependence accompanying a brief illness disappears with the return of physical vigor, but a long or indefinite one accompanying a chronic state of ill health may mean difficult adjustment.

Some persons, forced by illness to be dependent upon others, become irritable, or withdrawn, or stubborn and unable to carry out suggestions. Others luxuriate in the opportunity to be dependent, becoming demanding, whining, bafflingly unable to get well. Fortunately, most persons are only as emotionally dependent as they need to be physically—allowing a suitable margin for individual background.

It is important for the worker to be certain in her own mind about the naturalness and inevitability of the sick person's need to lean, to accept it and to know that it must be met by someone and, preferably, by several persons. When the normal need is met through physical care and through the interest of physician, family or family substitute, church, friends, minister, volunteers, nurse, and a reliable, interested social worker, the client can use to the maximum the opportunities he has to improve physically. Unmet psychological needs are not added to the physical burden with which he must cope. As soon as physical strength permits, maximum independence, activity, effort, and concern for others may need to be encouraged.

THE FAMILY

One cannot separate consideration of the client from that of his family. They influence him constantly, physically and emotionally. The disabling illness which has changed his life has also changed theirs. When his usual role changed, theirs likewise did. If, for example, a mother who was the pivot of family life is either removed to a hospital or is preoccupied with pain and physical incapacity, a disequilibrium results until others in the family take over some of her duties and learn to get along without her comfort and guidance.

How well the family weathers the strain and regroups itself depends upon many things. Often a spouse, who formerly leaned on the one who is now invalid and upon whom much additional work and worry have fallen, needs to secure from someone else the emotional support he or she formerly had from the invalid.

The worker needs to be perceptive of what is happening in the family, quietly observing and aware of the remarks that are made. If the spouse follows the worker out to the car, or makes excuses to telephone her, or to come into the office, this may be the worker's cue to take the time to listen, to give a little encouragement, and to convey the assurance that someone understands.

When it seems that the spouse is going to need substantial moral support and a chance to unburden for a long period of time, the worker will need to decide whether she can try to meet this need or whether there is someone else who is in a better position to do so. Sometimes a potentially helpful relative may be the answer if any existing problems, such as transportation, can be overcome. In some instances, a clergyman can be alerted to the need.

When children are deprived of the companionship and guidance of the sick person, and the well parent is overburdened with worry, they may need extra attention from relatives, school personnel, Sunday school teacher, Boy Scout troop leader, or whoever may be available.

Most important is the gradual return of the sick or disabled person to maximum family participation. Physical invalids can still function as strong family members if they are not in constant pain, as few are, or are not in a terminal state. The more the sick person feels an important part in the family, the better off he is, and the less adjustment the rest of the family must make.

The Physician

Because the physician's ministrations may be lifesaving, he symbolizes an authority rarely equaled by men in other capacities. Hence, patients, social workers, and others may fail to think of him objectively. The patient and the social worker may mentally associate him with characteristics he does not possess but which they unconsciously vest in authority. These may be characteristics of exceeding virtue or of lack of worth, depending upon the experiences the individual patient or worker may have had with authoritative figures.

For these and other reasons, social workers either seem excessively to dislike and fear all physicians or to think that anything a doctor says is infallible and not to be questioned. The public welfare worker cannot afford either of these distortions.

Doctors may have equally distorted misapprehensions about social workers, associating us with socialized medicine or thinking of us as either hard-boiled snoopers or fuzzy-minded dreamers.

It is of the greatest consequence to the client that social workers individualize physicians as we do everyone else, that we think and act realistically in relation to each of them, and that we make a conscious effort to work effectively with them in behalf of sick or disabled clients.

Getting acquainted is the first step. This means taking the time for an office visit to the physician (by appointment), especially at first, instead of using a telephone call or letter to secure information. As the doctor learns that we are genuinely interested in helping his patient, our client, to overcome the social obstacles that stand in the way of his greatest possible recovery, he usually becomes an ally and friend. We must demonstrate through our actions that we can be trusted with medical information and that we are intelligently interested in learning as much as we can.

Physicians who work in hospitals that provide free care to the indigent often work under unusual handicaps. Depending upon the size of the hospital, its accreditation and staffing pattern, many of the doctors are interns and residents. Interns frequently "rotate" from one service to another in a hospital, sometimes as often as every three weeks in a large hospital, in order to secure at least a glimpse of the various kinds of medical problems. A continuing relationship with any one patient, or a comprehensive knowledge of the patient's social problems, personality, and total response to illness, may be almost impossible. Interns work under extraordinary pressure in many hospitals with a back-breaking burden of responsibility for details. Many interns therefore do not have the time or opportunity to respond to inquiries in the way a social worker would like.

An intern who decides to specialize may become a resident for three to five years. A "first-year resident" may be an inexperienced person (although this is not always true) whereas a chief resident, someone in his last year of specialty training and selected as chief because of demonstrated capacity, may be highly qualified. Residents have in common a desire to learn from their hospital experience as much as possible, so that the patients who have complicated medical problems are more interesting to them than the individuals with long-time chronic disease.

Frequently residents want to deal with a variety of different problems, in order to widen their scope of knowledge, and this can influence them toward early discharge of the patient, especially if there is a waiting list for hospital beds. Residents are usually not so hard-pressed as interns, but in hospitals which have an insufficient number of "visiting" or "attending" staff (full-fledged physicians who usually give their time free to a municipal or county hospital), the residents also may be extremely busy persons.

Although institutions which provide free care differ, the medical staff cannot usually be expected to give much time to any one clinic patient, and the rotation in staff on different services frequently prevents them from gaining the personal knowledge of the patient's problems and reactions which is ideal. The patient may have no opportunity for a relationship with one physician. Social workers may therefore have to take initiative in helping the client who is a clinic patient to secure the information he needs, and to give him much support.

Generally, we can expect the greatest interest in the patient from the family physician who has known and cared for him for some time. He can be counted on more than the specialist who sees the client only once or the shifting members of a clinic staff.

Of the specialists, internists (sometimes called diagnosticians) are, along with pediatricians, usually most interested in the social needs of their patients and are thus most able to be of help to the social worker.

In working with physicians, we should avoid those things that commonly make them impatient with us. Doctors are frequently busy and harassed; we need to be considerate of their time and to get to the point. They need to know *why* we want to know; otherwise they may think that giving us information about their patients is a violation of their ethics.

Doctors cringe when lay persons try to make diagnoses; we unconsciously do this more often than we realize. For example, the social worker may say, "This child has tonsillitis," or "This child needs his tonsils out," instead of merely, "This child has a sore throat." Doctors may also cringe when lay persons use medical terms; this may seem to them an invasion of their world. It is better to use lay language.

As is true in any relationship, a general knowledge of and interest in the other person's field makes communication possible. That is, the worker needs to be able to respond intelligently to the doctor's remarks, and to ask relevant questions. Groundwork for communication comes from reading the readily available material on medical subjects in magazines and newspapers and watching television shows about medicine. Referring to a medical dictionary, conferring with the agency medical consultant whenever indicated and according to the possibilities in the agency, learning common medical prefixes and suffixes, are all ways in which the worker can improve her capacity to ask the right questions and to respond intelligently when working with the client's physician.

One of the problems social workers occasionally encounter among physicians is an adverse personal reaction toward the client or an attitude of impatience and severity regarding his behavior. The doctor may reflect certain widely held community attitudes that assistance recipients are shiftless and somehow beneath the self-supporting population.

If such an attitude seems to exist and to stand in the way of good planning in the client's behalf, the worker may be able to modify the physician's attitude by giving him brief and pertinent information about the client's situation. An understanding of the client's problems will often change an initially adverse reaction. The worker has an obligation to her client to emphasize the positive, so far as this is honest, and not to reinforce the negative about him.

Sharing social information with the physician should be done with relevance to the medical problem and to the physician's concern. For example, a doctor may be impatient with a diabetic who fails to stay on his diet. If the social worker knows that the diabetic's wife is blind, or that he receives surplus commodities only, or that the wife has been unable to secure an appointment with the dietitian, she should describe briefly whatever extenuating circumstances exist. The worker may soon find that the physician will become more interested in the client and anxious to help him. The worker should exert special care not to present irrelevant material, however interesting it may seem, which merely takes the doctor's time and does not illuminate the medical-social problems.

Other Colleagues

In working with the sick or disabled, the social worker is only one of a group of helping persons, because there are many things the client needs which are outside the competence of a social worker. Just as the physician plays a vital role in the client's life, so may the visiting nurse, the vocational rehabilitation counselor, the minister, the dietitian, and sometimes the physical and occupational therapist. It takes more time to work with others, but much more can be accomplished and sometimes it saves time in the end.

THE PUBLIC HEALTH NURSE

The public health nurse's primary function is individualized health teaching. She usually does not take on continuing nursing duties, as the private visiting nursing agency sometimes does, but she will often demonstrate to some member of the family how to take care of the patient. If a client is bedfast or chair bound, he greatly needs the kind of help a public health nurse can give in suggesting home modifications that will make his care easier and more scientific, and in helping the family give care which will prevent needless disability from bedsores, deformities, bowel and bladder complications, and other upsets. Public health and private visiting nurses will usually make only one visit without a doctor's order. They are better able than the welfare worker to learn from the physician what care he wants performed. However, if the worker is talking with the physician, it is well to ask him if he thinks it would be a good idea to ask a nurse to go to the home to teach the family how to give nursing care to the patient.

Public health nurses are occasionally so busy conducting well-baby clinics and following up on communicable disease cases that the social worker hesitates to ask the nurse to visit an adult who is ill or disabled. Most health departments are understaffed and their nurses overworked. Chronic disease is, however, an area appropriate to the health department's concern. If the health officer does not know the number of chronic disease cases, because no one brings the needs to his attention, he obviously has no ammunition to use on the board of supervisors toward securing a larger nursing staff. Therefore, even if a telephone call to the public health department brings no results for the client in question, it is constructive and worth taking the time to do. Many health departments have ruled against making home visits, again because of lack of nursing staff. The social worker does no harm in asking, and she may find to her surprise that the public health nurse can manage a call at the home of a patient when she is in the neighborhood or that she will make an exception.

THE VOCATIONAL REHABILITATION COUNSELOR

The vocational rehabilitation counselor is another busy but often vitally important person in the disabled client's life. He has at his command a variety of resources, and is often able to obtain physical treatment, equipment, and opportunities for the client which the worker is not. He is usually equipped to conduct simple psychological testing, and has a knowledge of industry that can greatly extend the social worker's ideas of possibilities for the client's adjustment and usefulness.

A rehabilitation agency is usually, like other community services, understaffed. Rehabilitation is an extremely slow, detailed, time-consuming process. Like most busy people, the counselor is likely to spend his time on the "coöperative" patient and on the person who has enough initiative to keep himself in the foreground of the counselor's mind. Therefore the social worker occasionally finds it necessary to do some prompting about her clients, and to perform the same kind of positive interpretation that is sometimes helpful with doctors and nurses.

THE CLERGYMAN

The priest, minister, or rabbi is an important colleague in services to the chronically ill. Religious consolation means more to those who are depressed, ill, and adjusting to severe limitations than the well commonly realize.

Nothing could be more unethical or distasteful than for a social worker to push her own religion with clients or to engage in theological discussions. She can, however, learn whether the client has been or is a church member, and whether he would like a clergyman to call. Clients whose church ties are weak or nonexistent may hesitate to take the initiative in developing a relationship with a church, or not know how, but respond with interest if the worker asks whether they would like to establish a church connection.

Clergymen, like doctors, deal with birth and death and are familiar with the sick room. Most of them relate easily and helpfully to sick persons. As with social workers, an occasional individual has an aversion to illness and finds it difficult to provide the amount of service desirable.

Social workers should acquaint themselves with the major distinguishing theological doctrines of the large denominations in order to know what philosophy to expect from various clergymen. For example, certain churches believe in the forgiveness of sin immediately upon repentance, which is helpful to some clients, whereas others are vague about the afterworld but emphasize goodness in this life.

Knowing the attributes of the outstanding clergymen in the community is helpful to the social worker who works with the ill or disabled. Some clergymen are especially interested in helping and are readily available, whereas others are burdened by mountainous duties in their parishes and less able to respond to the social worker's request for assistance.

THE CLINIC DIETITIAN

The clinic dietitian, or the nutritionist with a community agency, is of growing importance in work with the chronically ill because of the role of diet in medical treatment. Her specialized knowledge, translated into practical terms, may be literally lifesaving. The training of dietitians is, however, traditionally more in relation to feeding large groups of persons, as in hospitals or restaurants, than it is to helping individuals on low incomes to work out a special diet palatable to them. The worker may need to interpret the client's situation. The dietitian may not realize that he has limited cooking facilities or a limited educational background, or how low his food budget is.

The dietitian, because of her scientific training, is inclined to think in terms of grams and ounces and in scientific combinations of proteins, fats, and carbohydrates. Just as the worker needs to find out from the client, "What did the doctor tell you?" in order to get an impression of how much the client understands of his illness, she may need to ask "What did the dietitian have to say about your diet?" in order to find out whether the client needs a simpler or a repeated explanation.

PHYSICAL AND OCCUPATIONAL THERAPISTS

Physical and occupational therapists usually become well acquainted with their patients if they work with them for an extended period of time. Their ministrations encourage self-revelation, and they are usually interested in people. The therapist is a valuable colleague in securing a better understanding of the client's feelings and attitudes, as well as a source of information about his physical progress.

Occupational therapists may perform either "functional" or "recreational" therapy or both. The old role of the occupational therapist as someone who teaches the disabled person how to crochet to pass the time has generally changed to that of a person who helps the handicapped to learn self-care activities, such as how to use crippled hands to open a screen door, turn a door knob, comb hair, or put on shoes. Physical therapists perform the same type of duties as do occupational therapists in some communities, whereas in others the former concentrate largely on strengthening weakened muscles, teaching how to use crutches, and the like. One of the most valuable contributions these therapists make to the disabled person is to teach him how to make and use special devices or equipment.

Working with colleagues in behalf of a disabled person requires the sharing of information. Enough data must be given in conferences and confirming letters so that the others understand the client's realities and the problems he is going to face in carrying out medical recommendations or in coöperating in some plan for his rehabilitation. No danger exists that relevant information will be construed as gossip or as malicious in intent when it has been exchanged in a professional and constructive way for a purpose among persons accustomed to treating information confidentially. The danger comes when, in the heat of frustration over some particularly difficult or puzzling behavior, temptation exists to use the conference as a channel for releasing personal feelings or for sharing mutual feelings of inadequacy and anger.

When the client is intelligent and the subject can be introduced naturally, it is well to let him know that the worker proposes to attend a conference about his rehabilitation needs or about what other agencies can provide to be of help to him. He should be asked if there are matters or problems he feels should have particular emphasis. Clients are usually gratified to know that their situations are being given such conscientious and careful thought. The recipient should be informed about the results of the conference as soon as possible, and made to feel that his reactions are an important part of the total deliberation and planning—which they are, indeed.

How to Secure Information from a Hospital

Hospitals are special worlds geared to critical events moving at a fast tempo. Everything is subordinated to emergencies; when one acutely ill person becomes better, concern for him gives way to concern for another acutely ill person. After the former patient is discharged, he no longer exists for the personnel; they are absorbed in helping the new patient who now occupies the former's hospital bed.

The rapid tempo has greatly increased since the advent of "miracle drugs" and improvements in surgical techniques. The sick person recovers from his acute phase so rapidly that it seems he is no more than admitted when he is ready for discharge. Whereas the long process of recovery formerly permitted time for social planning while the person was in the hospital, now his bed is needed for the new patient before the gears can mesh between hospital and agency personnel.

The cost of each hospital day is so great and the need for the beds so urgent that severe pressure exists to discharge the patient as quickly as his physical condition permits. Room for friction between hospital and social agency personnel exists because the social worker cannot drop everything else on the instant the hospital telephones; if the public assistance worker is slow in responding, the hospital worker feels caught in a vise between the pressures of the hospital and the social agency's inability to act.

The long, slow progression of chronic disease cannot compete in medical fascination with the dramatic responses of the acutely ill. Therefore the chronic disease patient who "ties up a bed" may seem especially irksome to the busy resident in charge of a county hospital ward. His pressure on the hospital social worker to get the patient out may therefore be especially intense.

To be forewarned is to be forearmed. As soon as the worker knows that a client is in the hospital, telephone inquiry should be made of the hospital social worker (if the hospital has one) about the recipient's condition, whether change in living plans may be necessary upon discharge, and how quickly discharge may be anticipated. The client's pressing social problems, his current living arrangements, and provisions for care and supervision at home should be relayed. The worker should advise as to what her telephone hours are and how best to reach her.

The hospital worker, having been alerted to the existence of the patient and of his social situation, can then inquire of the physician what the patient's physical condition is and what the expected course will be. By no means will the physician always be able to make an accurate prediction, but he will know from the beginning that a social agency is interested, will know something about the patient's social situation, and will be much more likely to provide helpful information in advance of discharge than if no inquiry had been made. The hospital social worker will have been involved in the case early, and thus, able to watch for developments, may ask questions on the ward and keep the social agency informed.

A good relationship between the hospital and welfare department is fostered by this kind of mutual alertness and interest in the recipient. Face-to-face conferences about especially difficult cases are particularly helpful in fostering mutual acquaintance, trust, and understanding. This builds a framework within which the public welfare worker can secure the information she needs in order to be helpful to the recipient after he leaves the hospital. It avoids the deadening situation whereby the worker routinely writes to the hospital asking for "diagnosis and prognosis" and after long delay receives information which may be difficult to understand and the relevance of which to social planning may be questionable.

If the hospital has no social worker, the public welfare worker is dependent upon the patient's physician for information. A family doctor treating a recipient in a private hospital is a good source of information; if the recipient is in a county hospital or teaching hospital, the senior resident in charge of the ward is usually the best person with whom to communicate by telephone. A request through the hospital social worker, individualized and framed in the context of why the worker needs to know and what she is especially interested in, should be made in writing or by telephone and confirmed in writing. If there is no hospital social worker who serves the clinics, the request should be made in writing of the hospital record room.

Asking the recipient to have the clinic doctor fill out a form ordinarily invites poor results. The doctor is so busy during clinic hours that he cannot stop and fill out a form; if he tucks it in his pocket, he may forget about it. Further, the physician in one clinic may not know about, or take responsibility for advising about, an even more serious or important condition being treated in another clinic in the same outpatient department.

CHAPTER II

The Psychosomatic Concept

POSSIBLY NO MEDICAL TERM is so widely misunderstood and misused as "psychosomatic." None has greater significance for social workers.

"Psyche" means "soul" or "mind"; "soma" "body." Together they form a word describing the unity and interrelationship of mind and body. Witness the hair stand up on a cat's back when a dog approaches, or the dilatation of a person's eyes when he sees something frightening. The psyche and the soma have interreacted, the organism responded as a whole. Recognition of this fact is so widespread that it has been incorporated in our very language: "She makes me sick," "he's a pain in the neck," "he makes my heart beat faster." The psychiatrists refer to this as "organ language."

The unified or psychosomatic response of the organism to every circumstance contains varying degrees of psyche and soma. Some responses are largely organic, others largely emotional; and there are all degrees between. One student facing a final examination cannot sleep; another has diarrhea; another cannot eat, or conversely has a great desire to eat; another is irritable and snaps at everyone; another grows quiet and absent-minded.

At this point in man's knowledge, we think that such conditions as pneumonia and cancer are largely caused by somatic factors, and that others such as stomach ulcers and certain skin disorders are largely the result of emotional upset or nerve strain. The causative factors in even these, which seem at opposite ends of the pole, are not clear-cut. The wide range between includes many diseases—such as rheumatoid arthritis, asthma, high blood pressure, and ulcerative colitis—which are thought to be caused by both organic and psychic factors, the admixture differing in different persons and the theory of causation varying according to different authorities.

The body reacts not only to the psyche but upon the psyche and the social situation. Consider the family disturbances which are the result of the hyperirritability of a mother with a thyroid condition; the "laziness" or seeming irresponsibility of a potential wage earner who fails in his duties because of undiagnosed undulant fever, malaria, hookworm, or anemia; the family problems which arise out of the emotionality of a stroke patient.

Then turn the coin and see the mental and physical disease caused by social problems: for example, the individuals, probably predisposed, who finally become psychotic after long rejection and frustration; or those who contract tuberculosis as a result of exposure to the germ and are subject to overcrowding, stress, and malnutrition.

"Psychosomatic" is an adjective referring to the comprehensive, or total, or interrelated relationship of mind and body. Man does not react in fragmentary fashion with separate entities, but as a unit. He reacts as a psycho-social-biological whole.

The meaning of "psychosomatic" seems so obvious that one wonders why it is widely misused. One cause for the confusion lies in the tendency to use the word interchangeably with "psychogenic" ("psyche" plus "genesis," or the Greek for "be born"). Many persons, even in educated circles, call psychogenic disturbances psychosomatic disease. This is incorrect literally, because all human responses are psychosomatic—that is, unified. To apply the term to diseases thought to be caused by emotion is to imply incorrectly, that no emotional component exists in other disease states.

Several disease conditions are, however, now thought to be psychogenic, or caused entirely or almost entirely by psychic factors. These include some of the serious neuroses which take a bodily form, such as conversion hysteria, sometimes called hysterical paralysis, in which the psychic maladjustment expresses itself as an actual paralysis. Some psychiatrists and other physicians also think that those diseases are psychogenic in which a substantial element of emotional causation exists, such as rheumatoid arthritis, stomach ulcers, asthma, high blood pressure, and ulcerative colitis.

Psychogenic disease also includes cases in which symptoms appear that are similar to those caused by a diseased organ; the symptoms are, however, created by the improper function—not disease—of the organ. The action of the hypothalamus and the autonomic nervous system create malfunctioning in response to distressing emotion. For example, a gall bladder may stop functioning because of a squeezing of the duct from nervous tension, causing the same results as if a stone blocked the duct. Similar conditions, often called functional, are literally psychogenic.

The main reason why "psychosomatic" is misused or misunderstood is that many persons fail to understand the physiology of functional or psychogenic pain and consider it imaginary. In other words, they confuse it with malingering (outright lying) or at least with hypochondriasis (exaggeration of symptoms).

Thus, one sometimes hears "psychosomatic" used as a contemptuous derogation, or to mean "mere" or "inconsequential." Some social workers tend to make self-diagnoses or to diagnose clients or others as having psychosomatic disease—a dangerous practice indeed.

Practical Application

An understanding of psychosomatic relationships is of practical importance to all who work with human beings. Authors vary in their estimates, but it has been said that as much as three-fourths of medical practice is in behalf of persons needing care because of illness with a large emotional component.

Medical treatment often fails unless social and emotional problems which impede recovery are overcome. The convalescence of a worried person is notoriously slow; the danger inherent in operating upon a seriously frightened or disturbed person is well known in medical circles; the precipitating effect of emotional upsets upon certain diseases, such as arthritis or diabetes, is equally well known.

One aspect of psychosomatic relationships widely recognized among our associates, but seemingly forgotten at times about clients, is that physical distress or debility has emotional consequences. Severe or prolonged illness causes childishness, preoccupation with self, and emotional dependency. The long-time sufferer may become demanding or hostile as a normal consequence of his illness. Those who fail to recognize that sick people need to lean, or who forget that everyone wants to "talk about his operation," may condemn the individual as a complainer or ridicule his preoccupation with symptoms.

In those cases in which severe neuroses underlie the physical problems, the public assistance worker can do little to change the situation other than to collaborate with the physician in referring the client to a psychiatrist. However, the origin of the emotional upset is often found in social circumstances which the social worker can change or in misapprehension which the physician can rectify if he knows what the client is worried about.

Consequently it is important for all social workers, whatever their caseloads, to know that psychogenic pain or distress can be as severe as organic pain; to understand what "psychosomatic" means; to expect emotional problems when physical illness exists; and, if the psychic disturbance is socially caused, to take appropriate steps to reduce it.

Every sick person deserves a thorough physical examination and a sufficient period of observation before organic disease is ruled out. The anxieties and infantilism created by pain or infection are literally psychosomatic, but they are best reduced by provision of medical treatment and good physical care.

General Medical Base for Social Planning

HISTORICAL EVOLUTION

The medicine men of earliest times, being ignorant of any other approach, treated man as a unit of body and mind. "Modern" medicine, at its inception in ancient Greece, also considered man as a whole. After the Renaissance and the slow emergence of the scientific era in medicine, the old wisdom was lost in the whirlwind of gains, especially those of this century.

Slowly, interest in man as a whole being emerged again from different directions. The physiologists, experimenting on animals, showed how dogs and cats reacted bodily to rage, fear, pain, and hunger. Medical social workers in hospitals repeatedly pointed out the correlation of stress and illness. Psychiatry, particularly psychoanalysis, contributed greatly to an understanding of the psychosomatic concept. The idea that man, or the organism, functions as a unit of mind, body, and environment became the subject of exhaustive study and formidable terms.

Finally, the research which resulted in the use of ACTH and cortisone for arthritis elucidated and publicized the methods the body uses to respond to emotions. Thus, in the last two decades the full arc of the circle has been joined —from primitive medicine man to modern biochemist— in considering man as a whole.

THE HYPOTHALAMUS

A rational basis for understanding the unified or psychosomatic approach to the human organism begins with an acquaintance with the hypothalamus. This is a part of the brain which is the control center for the bodily expression of emotion or for the reception and integration of responses associated with fear and rage.

Sensory pathways lead to the hypothalamus, flashing images from the environment which carry connotations of danger or any other form of emotional excitation. The hypothalamus then musters the appropriate bodily responses to rise to the occasion. (In passing, it should be noted that something which creates an old memory of danger or anger arouses reactions of anxiety to a greater or less degree in the same physiological manner as a present danger.)

The hypothalamus operates first upon the master gland —the pituitary—and through it on the adrenal cortex, which is the outside cover of small glands above the kidneys. The adrenal cortex sends out substances that influence a large number of body functions, such as the circulatory and respiratory systems, sexual activities, and carbohydrate and fat metabolism. The hypothalamus also determines body temperature and the sleep function.

The hypothalamus operates not only by way of the glands but also through the autonomic (sometimes called vegetative) nervous system. This is a separate nervous system which has a network of nerves, connected to the spinal cord, that sends out an extended network of fibers to the organs of the abdomen and pelvis and the so-called smooth muscles.

These nerves dilate the eyes, moisten the skin with perspiration, send blood to heart and skeletal muscles, and generally prepare the body for "fight or flight." They create the sensations and the reactions that accompany the emotions, and are not under the control of the conscious will.

Nature gave man this intricate response to stress to permit him to protect himself from danger by quick and automatic reactions. However, if the stress mechanism is called upon constantly or for too long, this protective equipment backfires and health is undermined.

THE MEANING OF STRESS

Many stress experiments have been conducted on animals and men. Observation and interviews have shown that the stress a person is under and his individual way of mastering it are major factors affecting his health.

Stress results from infection, injuries, shock, heat or cold, hunger, and nervous strain. According to Hans Selye, the foremost physiological investigator of the subject, the reaction to stress is a physiological "alarm reaction" or adaptation response. When the stress continues for a long period, the response mechanisms become exhausted, and this exhaustion can cause damage to the tissues. The "stressors" are perceived and acted upon by the hypothalamus and the autonomic nervous system, as indicated previously.

Further experiments show that in nerve strain it is not the event that determines the stress reaction but the way in which the individual reacts to the event. Some persons react violently to certain events, some not at all. Of those who react, some master their emotions by "getting them out of their systems." Others are unable to master the upset state of mind—the disturbance smolders or festers; these are the persons most likely to become seriously affected.

Why are some persons unable to react outwardly to feelings of frustration and outrage? The way of reacting is determined by early family relationships: whether a child grew up with a secure or a fearful concept of himself, whether he dared show hostile feelings or was so frightened by unloving or unstable parents that he had to develop a pattern of curbing expressions of emotions.

Giving an individual an opportunity to express his emotions over frustrating or threatening or frightening events helps him to avoid later harmful bodily effects from the experience. The way one person reacts to a situation is not an indication of how another will.

People are emotionally vulnerable to different situations, depending upon significant experiences in their early lives. For example, to have his assistance check held may not particularly affect one person, whereas another may feel humiliated and angry. Of those who feel especially upset, some will be afraid to express their feelings or totally unable to express them. The latter are those who may have psychosomatic effects from the experience.

Implications for Public Assistance

The implications of the psychosomatic concept of illness are wide for public assistance. The everyday social problems of hunger, cold, fear, severe strain, and disease are stressors. Prolonged stress causes illness; illness in turn causes stress. Not surprisingly, we are concerned with generations of dependents, with multiproblem families, and with illness as the most costly aspect of public assistance.

The implications of the psychosomatic concept may be divided into the broad preventive aspects, the general ameliorative aspects, and the specific application in working with individual sick persons.

PREVENTION

As so often happens in considering problems of human behavior, we are forced back to the importance of the prenatal period and early life of the child. Some pregnant women have such excessive burdens that they cannot welcome a coming child. They do not have psychic energy available to love him when he arrives. By helping such a woman lessen her social problems, so that she has more energy to give to her child, a worker can indirectly help the child form the foundation for personality which tolerates stress well in later life. Such simple measures as providing repairs for a broken washing machine or arranging day nursery care for noisy active toddlers can contribute to this goal.

An examination of public assistance procedures shows

the amount of work ahead of us in arriving at practical ways
to achieve these ends. Federal participation in general assistance may prove a great stimulus toward policies which
will make it possible for some unemployed fathers who now
desert to remain with their families. If mothers receiving
aid for dependent children can be less harassed by investi-
gators and by guilt over antisocial methods designed to
provide food and recreation, they will have more of themselves to give their children. When we can view rehabilitation not as forcing a mother to work to get off relief but
as help in alleviating crippling behavior, we can look for
more security in children.

However, social workers and their administrators cannot wait for these better days before taking constructive
steps. Vital measures toward accomplishing these goals are:
reduced caseloads and work simplification, more academic
and inservice training, and especially the provision of supervision which strengthens positive attitudes.

Administration must face the fact that enormous demands
are placed upon workers, including emotionally traumatiz-
ing and conflict-producing demands. The supervisor who can
absorb the resultant disturbance and hostility with equanimity and give acceptance and wise guidance in return is a
person of rare capacity. Yet these supervisors do exist in
county welfare departments, and their number needs to be
expanded through recognition, provision for training, and
reduction in pressures upon them.

GENERAL AMELIORATION

Minimizing stress of all kinds and affording a climate in
which the recipients under emotional tension can relieve
this form of stress are goals involving all workers. It will
be recalled that prolonged stress can cause illness and that

inability to express frustration and anger are also conducive to disease.

Adequate financial assistance, administered ungrudgingly and for a sufficient length of time so that the individual knows security, is a practical means of relieving many stress situations. The benefit is nullified if checks are frequently held up for recomputation of small amounts of income; if special need verifications are required which are difficult or humiliating for the clients to secure; if clothing may be purchased only after exhausting pricing effort; or, in other words, if our procedures are conducive to resentment and insecurity.

There are times in a large agency when necessary procedures are not well adapted to the needs of certain clients. The worker may regret this deeply, or even feel annoyed at her agency, but be unable to do anything to change the situation. This calls for delicate handling.

The worker should be permissive with the client, and conceal any negative feelings of her own so that she neither reinforces the client's anger nor retaliates against him for it (both equally destructive). She should try to let the client get his problem out into the open, and help him see that his frustration is the result of an unfortunate reality that cannot be changed by the welfare department. If the client can do this and still feel that he is understood and liked in spite of having blown off steam, the worker has ameliorated stress.

Much stress is environmental and of the kind which the worker can frequently help alleviate: poor living conditions, inadequate protection from cold, toothaches, earache, constant colds, inadequate laundry facilities, not enough clothes. An endless list of human stresses is so commonplace to the public assistance worker that her worst enemy is getting so accustomed to them that she sees them no longer. If seen, many problems can be remedied through the grant, medical care, and community resources. The relationship built up as a by-product of persistent mutual effort by worker and client to alleviate his stress is an additional source of healing to the client.

APPROACH TO THE SICK PERSON

Having glimpsed the magnitude and pervasiveness of psychosomatic relationships, we find it inconceivable that anyone could use the term "psychosomatic" as a synonym for "mere," or "imaginary," or as contemptuous derogation.

Recalling, however, how widespread the misconceptions are, we are not surprised that even an occasional physician may misuse the term or confuse it with malingering or with moral weakness. The client may smart with resentment and a sense of injustice if no organic disease is held accountable for his pains or distress. This is particularly true if the patient feels that the physician has been curt with him.

The client deserves an adequate interpretation of his illness from his physician; the social worker is not the person to explain that his illness is caused or aggravated by stress. However, if the client has come from an examination frustrated and angry or let down and upset because he has been led to believe that the doctor "found nothing wrong with me," or that the doctor "said it was all in my head," then the worker has an obligation to find out from the doctor just what he believes the situation to be and what the client was told.

If possible, the client should return to the doctor for an interview with additional explanations and a chance to ask questions. If this is not possible, the worker may elaborate on what the doctor has already told the client and help him differentiate between malingering and psychogenic illness.

She may help him accept the fact that "nerves" can be as powerful as organic injury in creating pain and malfunction, and that the physiological effect is complex but not mysterious.

If the client has had a thorough physical examination, and the doctor finds that the symptoms are greater than organic findings would indicate, the worker should examine the social situation with the client to see whether obvious forms of social stress exist. Efforts directed toward environmental improvement or improvement in family relationships will usually require continued work for a period of time.

A true neurosis, such as conversion hysteria, expressed as a physical condition—that is, an illness which is considered entirely psychogenic (the diagnosis should be made by a psychiatrist)—will not usually yield to the efforts of the public assistance agency. Psychiatric assistance or that of a specially trained social worker is required. By no means will efforts of these highly equipped professional persons always result in a cure. The social worker should, however, coöperate with any such person treating the client, and help with the environmental problems within the welfare department's reach.

The same approach is required in organic illness—such as rheumatoid arthritis, asthma, essential hypertension, duodenal ulcers, and ulcerative colitis—in which psychic factors are thought to constitute an important underlying cause. These diseases must be attacked medically, which may include psychiatric participation if the attending physician so directs. The social worker's efforts should be directed toward relief of social stress that aggravates symptoms, interferes with medical treatment, or militates against rehabilitation.

Social work is as concerned with the emotional results of disease as with emotional aspects of causation. Dependency induced by illness, discussed in Chapter I, probably constitutes the major problem.

Of first importance is understanding one's own reaction to dependency. Most persons seem to dislike having others lean on them, and either try to avoid the dependent person or may even be tempted, unconsciously, to retaliate against him. Because the tendency must be avoided, we can lessen the dependency upon ourselves by arranging for friendly visitors or others, such as clergymen and nurses, to share a part of it, as previously discussed. More important, we can help strengthen the person emotionally through trying to see that medical care problems are solved, meeting legitimate social needs ungrudgingly, concentrating with the client, when it is natural and opportune, on the situations in his life when he functioned well and independently.

CHAPTER III

Rheumatoid Arthritis

ARTHRITIS is a formidable disease, generally conceded to be responsible for more crippling than any other. The two most common kinds are rheumatoid arthritis and osteo-arthritis. The latter is the "gray hair of the bones," present in some degree in most older persons and sometimes responsible for severe disability in the aged. This chapter will discuss only rheumatoid arthritis, which is the progressive, severely crippling form that usually comes to mind when arthritis is mentioned.

Rheumatoid arthritis is predominantly a disease of early middle age. It does occur in children (called *Still's disease*), but begins most frequently around the age of thirty-five. More women than men have rheumatoid arthritis of the extremities; more men than women have the spinal form (usually called *spondylitis* or *Marie Strumpell's disease*).

Assistance planning should be thought of from the beginning in terms of the appropriate categorical aids rather than in terms of short-time or emergency relief, not because the client may never be able to go back to work but because of the length of time involved and because medical treatment and maximum prevention of deformities require rest and, frequently, occupational change.

General Medical Base for Social Planning

CAUSE AND COURSE

The cause of rheumatoid arthritis is not known. Psychological factors are widely assumed to play a part. However, a recent evaluation of the literature reveals that most of the psychiatric studies have lacked adequate controls and therefore lack real scientific validity. The only corroborated psychological findings relate to the fact that most patients have an insecure background, many coming from broken homes.

In spite of lack of knowledge about the fundamental cause, physicians believe that stress of some kind (such as prolonged exposure to cold and damp, injury, pregnancy, infection, shock, worry) may precipitate rheumatoid arthritis in a person who suffers from chronic overfatigue. The disease begins in mechanically weak spots, that is, in joints which may have been subject to excessive abuse from occupational or other physical strain. Inflammation then occurs in the lining (*synovial membrane*), the capsule, and the tissue around the affected joints, causing pain and swelling.

The inflammation damages the cartilage at the ends of the two bones that form a joint. Unless this inflammation can be controlled, it will continue until the cartilage ulcerates and degenerates, causing a partial dislocation (*subluxation*) or the two bones to become fused or permanently stiffened (*ankylosed*).

The stress not only causes the tissue reaction to occur in one or more joints but triggers a total bodily reaction which causes muscle spasm and wasting, excessive fatigue, anemia, loss of weight, and a general sense of malaise. These symptoms may be accompanied by stomach or heart trouble and a variety of other bodily ailments.

In the earliest stages of the disease, the joint pain and swelling are usually fleeting and may disappear entirely for months or years at a time. Usually the disease returns; each time it does, the active stage lasts longer, more joints are involved, and more joint damage and muscle wasting occur.

An arthritic individual who after a long period of active disease arrives at a static crippled condition in which he has no pain is sometimes referred to as a "burned-out" arthritic. Authorities point out that the term is a misnomer, for although the active process seems to have disappeared completely, it may return. Arthritis, in other words, is never considered cured.

EFFECTS OF THE DISEASE

The pain of rheumatoid arthritis, which may be constant or intermittent, severe or slight, is, along with deformity, the major characteristic which differentiates it from other long-time crippling conditions.

The cerebral palsied person, for example, can confine his battle to overcoming the tremendous frustrations imposed by the refusal of his body to do his bidding. But the arthritic has to fight pain as well—long-lasting, enervating, nerve-wracking pain, from which he may or may not have periods of relief. Not only does long-continued pain have disabling effects on the personality; pain also interferes with rehabilitation, because it limits the exercising of joints and the self-care adaptations which are part of physical restoration. The pain is present while the disease process is active, and is accentuated when stretching of stiffened joints and muscles is attempted.

Deformities occur in several ways. When the joint linings swell and scarring occurs, a partial dislocation may finally take place and distortions occur. Muscles shrink and become weakened, and incorrect balance in the bending and extending effects of muscle pairs creates mechanical problems. The lack of use of the muscles creates a vicious-circle effect. Finally, deformity occurs because the person adopts fixed positions which provide the greatest comfort. He instinctively carries his arms, bends his legs, sits, or lies in positions which minimize the pain. These positions of the extremities eventually become fixed. Thus in the early stages of the disease it is important for the patient to have professional advice about positioning and sometimes to be placed in corrective casts or splints.

If a person is working at a job which requires the same muscle and joint positions, as most labor does, the occupation itself contributes to the deformity. Change of occupation is thus often necessary. Sitting in a chair that is too low, lying on a soft mattress, using pillows incorrectly, and lying in the wrong position are some of the other everyday ways in which deformities are unwittingly created.

Most important, deformities become permanent if the abnormal positions are permitted to remain fixed long enough, but can be minimized if intelligent, comprehensive treatment is begun soon enough. Thus, whether the apparent crippling is reversible or irreversible is an extremely important diagnostic point in medical and social planning. The deformities may look permanent, and the individual may be unable to bend the joint, but permanent joint destruction still may not have occurred. This can be determined only by X ray. Even in a neglected case, treatment may still be started in time to save the client from undue disabling deformities.

When an individual has a disease which weakens him, makes him feel miserable, and causes acute pain, he cannot be expected to use normal initiative. Social workers frequently find arthritics hostile or distant and reluctant to talk about themselves. Arthritics often have marital problems. Whether these things are a result of their physical condition is a moot point, but it is logical to think that adverse social and psychological effects would come about from the weakness, malaise, and prolonged pain which are a part of this disease.

TREATMENT

There is no specific cure for rheumatoid arthritis. The aims of treatment are to relieve symptoms and prevent further crippling. About 50 per cent of the cases are said to respond to conservative measures. *Treatment must be begun at the earliest possible moment,* and this does not refer to an occasional visit to a doctor or to casual or sporadic attention at the county hospital clinic. Untold sums of public money and of human suffering are at stake in getting the rheumatoid arthritic under thorough, comprehensive treatment as soon as he comes to the attention of the welfare department. Treatment is often expensive. However, years of institutional care for the needlessly permanently deformed arthritic are even more expensive.

Treatment may require the help of the social worker as well as the doctor, because much of it is aimed at improving the general bodily condition. Attention is given to rest, weight gain, improved nutrition, and frequently to the intake of Vitamins A, B, C, and D. Warmth is also important, which creates an exacting housing requirement.

Many different kinds of drugs are used to relieve pain

and bring the disease process under control. These range from massive doses of aspirin to gold therapy, fever therapy, vaccines, thyroid and hormonal extracts, and in recent years to ACTH and the other so-called *steroids* (cortisone and similar drugs). Many of the powerful drugs are potentially dangerous, and it is essential that the patient stay under close medical supervision while he is taking them.

The steroids are often dramatic in bringing about temporary relief from the pain and crippling effects of arthritis. They are expensive, but in light of the extraordinary effects they have on many patients they may be well worth the price. However, if the person must have large doses in order to get relief, he will be subject to possible serious side effects and will need careful watching by the physician. Further, when the drugs are discontinued, the patient may get worse than he was originally. The physician must determine whether he thinks it worth while to try one of the steroids on the patient and take the risk. If he does, every effort should be made to finance the client's treatment and also to make certain that the client is seeing the doctor regularly.

From the social worker's point of view, one of the most important aspects of treatment is that the convalescing arthritic is in a precarious state of balance and needs a certain amount of protection. Little things may undo all the gains made and start him downhill again. Overdoing, emotional upsets, cold, hunger, infection, or any other form of stress is hazardous to the state of balance.

Careful management of exercise by physician and physiotherapist is another essential in treatment. One often hears that arthritics "should keep going." This is true, but the individual needs the right kind and amount of exercise to keep his muscles in tone without fatiguing him. Overuse of an inflamed joint will create destruction of bone surfaces, and then they may grow together permanently. The right balance between rest and exercise must be prescribed by the physician. The patient must be conscientious in stopping his activity before the point of fatigue or pain and in alternating activity with rest.

Surgery is sometimes employed to correct deformities, especially in the hips, knees, and elbows, but is usually not performed until the active disease process has disappeared. *Arthroplasty* (plastic surgery to restore movement to the joint), *arthrodesis* (repair of a deformity and stiffening of a joint in a more desirable position for occupation or stability), and *synovectomy* (removal of an affected membrane in a joint) are the common forms of surgery used. These operations must be carried out by experienced orthopedic specialists, and are said to be at least partly successful in most of the relatively few cases where they can be performed.

Other forms of treatment include the application of casts or splints, and manipulation (forceful straightening) under anesthesia. In most cases, however, the arthritic is helped by long-time conservative treatment—that is, by medical supervision, drugs, and careful attention by the client and his social worker, physical therapist, and public health nurse to the practical aspects of his daily regimen and environment. Enough rest, the right shoes, a chair of the right height, a bed board under the mattress, warm clothing, adequate housing, and good nutrition are essential aids to adequate medical care.

Implications for Public Assistance

Rheumatoid arthritis by no means always progresses to extreme disability. It is unpredictable in that some persons have long periods of remission or abatement and others have short ones. Unpredictability causes problems in itself, and arthritis is a long-time disruptive condition, eventually creating the necessity of a whole new adaptation to life for the family as well as for the patient.

If case classification is used or a similar method of sorting out cases needing intensive work, clients with this disease should be placed in the group to which most attention is to be given, because medical treatment contains such a large social component. When the budget is set up or revised, the maximum permissible for housing and utilities should be allowed, warmth and constant temperatures being vital, as has been pointed out. The same is true of the food budget because of the importance of nutrition.

REST

Rest, a vital matter in the treatment of rheumatoid arthritis, is one of the most difficult recommendations to carry out. Doctors often fail to give sufficiently specific orders, and the patient does not know how long he is to rest, whether he is to go to bed, sit in a chair, or just what he is to do. The homemaker may see the housework pile up, and have children who need her active assistance or intervention. The man may feel guilty lying around the home having to accept relief while his family does without many things they need. The worker, naturally eager to rehabilitate her clients and see them off the assistance rolls, may not feel that she should discourage attempts at employment.

Rest may not mean complete inactivity, and limited employment is frequently permissible. Therefore the worker and the recipient must secure clear and explicit recommendations from the physician as to the amount of rest, the kind, and for how long.

CHARACTERISTIC NEEDS

Items frequently needed include high-protein, high-caloric diet (a bland diet may also be prescribed at times), orthopedic shoes, blankets, hot water bottles or heating pads, heaters, and chair adaptations permitting the client to sit at the correct height. Provision may also be needed for a hard but comfortable mattress and bed board.

Depending upon the client's condition and deformities, there may also be needed: canes and crutches, a wheel chair or chair with casters, ramps, bars in the bathroom, elevated toilet seat, and the great variety of other devices which improve self-care, avoid strain on inflamed joints, and decrease the burden on the family. Through the pamphlets of the Arthritis and Rheumatism Foundation, ideas can be found for manifold ingenious devices which help the client in such activities as dressing, bathing, and using toilet facilities. Many of these devices can be homemade or worked out by a mechanically minded relative or volunteer.

TRANSPORTATION

Transportation to the clinic or doctor's office often proves one of the most difficult social obstacles to medical treatment. If because of his degree of disability the client cannot use public transportation, provision must be made for either automobile or taxi rides. Because the arthritic client is highly motivated to get rid of his pain he can be counted on to do everything in his power while he thinks the treatment will do him some good, but when the long discouraging stage sets in he may need a good deal of help and encouragement. Transportation needs to be made as easy as possible for him. At best, getting to the doctor's office is going to be painful and a clinic visit is usually exhausting.

COUNSELING

Because psychogenic factors are thought to be important, but because deep psychotherapy is frequently not practical, supportive help is as much as can be provided in most circumstances. As the client may well have been an unusually hard-working person, and also may be essentially insecure, it is apparent that the adjustment to long-time semi-invalidism or complete invalidism will be difficult for him.

Family relationships frequently change when the homemaker or breadwinner is no longer able to play his accustomed role. Divorce or separation seems frequent where arthritis exists, probably to some extent because the patient cannot play his expected role in family life. A homemaker or part-time housekeeping help will assist in keeping the woman client's family together, by preventing undue, prolonged burden on the husband and children. Giving the spouse a chance to talk out his troubles and helping as much as possible may prevent family breakup. A consistent social plan, with the minimum of insecurities, is important.

Although a Pollyannish attitude will only serve to make the client feel that his true condition is not understood, an attitude of pessimism or resignation is not warranted. Arthritics do get better, progressive deformity is not inevitable, and some even seem to become completely well for long periods of time. The worker should maintain a hopeful attitude.

In the fortunately infrequent cases of complete, permanent invalidism, institutional care may be necessary. There the individual is easily shelved or forgotten unless an effort is made by the worker to stimulate continued interest on the part of relatives, volunteers, and church contacts. Continued medical supervision, occupational therapy, and recreation (including television and reading materials) form the focus of other counseling efforts. The relationship developed between recipient and worker permits him to use her for as much release of feeling as he is able to express. Understanding, rather than false cheeriness, should be the worker's response.

REHABILITATION

Financing care at a rehabilitation center, after the client's disease process is under medical control, needs to be given thoughtful consideration if the crippling is extensive. Vocational rehabilitation may not be feasible, but improved self-care is an equally important goal. A medical evaluation of feasibility for rehabilitation is paramount, because the client may not be a good candidate physically. There is danger in beginning physical therapy too early. The family physician or internist in charge of the recipient should decide when physical restoration services should be considered. Ideally, the medical decision for physical restoration should be made jointly by a family doctor and an expert in physical medicine.

Vocational rehabilitation may be necessary for clients whose occupation was physically taxing. Immediate employment after improvement or remission of the disease is less important than preparation for employment which minimizes the likelihood of return of the disease or aggravation of crippling.

TERMS FREQUENTLY USED IN MEDICAL REPORTS

Acute infectious or **traumatic arthritis.** Rheumatoid arthritis caused by infection or injury.
Adduction contractures. Deformities in a drawn-up position.

Ankylosis. A permanent solid union of two bones at the joint.

Ankylosis spondylitis. Rheumatoid arthritis of the spine in which the vertebrae grow together, causing a "poker spine."

Arthralgia. Joint pain.

Arthro. Greek for "joint," the root in arthritic conditions.

Arthrodesis. Surgical stiffening of the joint sometimes resorted to in cases of uncontrollable pain or used to give stability.

Arthropathy. Joint disease.

Arthroplasty. Surgery of limited success designed to restore movement to a stiffened joint.

Atrophic. Wasting. Atrophic arthritis is a synonym for rheumatoid arthritis.

Bursitis. Inflammation of a bursa, which is a small sac filled with fluid to prevent friction of tissues which rub together.

Degenerative or hypertrophic arthritis. Osteoarthritis, the form to which old persons are subject.

Exacerbation. An aggravation or flare-up. The opposite of remission or abatement. The two are used together to describe ups and downs in disease, "exacerbations and remissions," as in rheumatoid arthritis.

Extension. An outright position.

Flexion. A bent position.

Fulminating. Severe, intense. Refers to an acute stage of disease.

Fusiform. Spindle-shaped.

Fusion. Same as *ankylosis*.

Herberden's nodes. Knobby lumps over finger joints; named for the physician who first described them.

Kyphosis. Hump or round curve of spine.

Marie Strumpell's disease. See *ankylosis spondylitis*.

Nonarticular. Not pertaining to a joint.

Osteo. *Greek* for "bone"; the root in all terms describing conditions of the bone.

Polyarthritis. Arthritis in more than one joint.

Rheumatoid spondylitis. See *ankylosis spondylitis*.

Sedimentation rate. A painless blood test which indicates whether there is active infection in the body.

Spondylitis rhizomelica. See *ankylosis spondylitis*.

Steroids. A group name for certain substances (for example, cortisone, prednisone) including some hormones, either naturally or artificially created, which affect various metabolic processes in the body. Those under discussion are used to heighten resistance.

Still's disease. Juvenile rheumatoid arthritis.

Subluxation. An incomplete or partial dislocation.

Synovial membrane. Lining of the joints, bursae, and tendon sheaths.

Synovial fluid. Produced by the synovial membrane, "oil for the hinge."

Tendo. Latin for "tendon."

Tendo- or **tenosynovitis.** Inflammation of the tendon sheaths.

CHAPTER IV

Diabetes Mellitus

DIABETES has such pervasive effects upon social adjustment that it is sometimes referred to as a way of life. The disease cannot be cured, but it can be controlled.

Most persons who maintain good control live satisfactory lives with only a moderate reduction in the average life span. If they do not achieve control, serious disability and death can result. Achieving control affects almost every aspect of the individual's life, from what and when he eats to the care he takes of his feet. In no disease does the outcome more directly depend upon the individual's own actions, emotions, and capacities. Like tuberculosis and heart disease, diabetes must be thought of as a medical-social, rather than as a strictly medical, problem.

Diabetes has increased to eighth place in 1957 as a major cause of death. The mortality rate has decreased among younger people, but is more prevalent among the elderly, and this segment of our population is, of course, growing.

White, overweight, married women are most subject to the disease. Approximately 50 per cent of diabetes is found in persons under fifty years of age, and, like cancer, it is often more severe in the young. In older persons, the hazards are primarily the result of the fact that diabetes is often accompanied by other diseases as well as by its own complications. Arteriosclerosis is common, with its foundations for gangrene, loss of sight, and heart disease.

The diabetic will be found in all aid programs, most frequently in those for the aged. Diabetics who have severe complications often qualify for programs for the disabled or blind.

General Medical Base for Social Planning

CAUSE

Diabetes is a disturbance of metabolism caused by an insufficient supply of insulin which is manufactured by the pancreas. Carbohydrates are not properly burned and used by the body. Free, unconverted sugar or glucose increases in the blood, and the body must call abnormally on other sources, notably fat, for energy. In the process, too much fat is released and excess products (*ketone bodies* or *acetone*) are set free in the blood. If this condition persists at a high level, *acidosis* occurs, which results in coma and death unless immediate treatment intervenes.

The reason for the breakdown in normal carbohydrate metabolism is complex and not entirely understood. An hereditary factor accounts for the frequency with which diabetes occurs in more than one member of the same family. Various endocrine glands other than the pancreas affect the metabolism including the pituitary, thyroid, and adrenal glands. Emotional stress is considered a precipitating factor in diabetes, perhaps owing to the way stress releases glandular substances into the blood stream.

Obesity is considered one of the most important factors in precipitating diabetes in a predisposed individual. Insulin supplies which are available to take care of normal food intake may not be sufficient to metabolize the excessive food intake which creates obesity. When a middle-aged or elderly overweight person reduces and stays on a proper diet, the diabetic manifestations frequently disappear.

Infections are also common predisposing factors. A cold or influenza may be the precipitant; tuberculosis has an especially bad effect on either the incipient diabetic or the person with established diabetes.

SYMPTOMS

The most common symptom of diabetes is the excretion of an abnormally large amount of urine (*polyuria*). Excessive thirst (*polydipsia*) may also occur and, in some cases, a striking increase in appetite (*polyphagia*). Weight loss and loss of strength are other symptoms which may make the person aware that something is wrong. An abnormal tendency to drowsiness after meals can also occur.

Not all diabetics have recognizable symptoms, so that some may go into coma before anyone discovers the cause. Death may occur because diagnosis and treatment cannot be secured quickly enough. In order to prevent such disastrous results, screening clinics which offer urinalysis and blood-sugar tests are set up in some cities. The routine urinalyses in connection with complete physical examinations and hospital admissions also serve as screening techniques.

CONTROL

Once a person has diabetes, the same things that can precipitate it in the first place can upset the control or balance which has been established by treatment. Treatment is essentially a matter of restricting carbohydrates and total food intake, and usually of giving insulin in the amount found necessary to metabolize the food. If too much or the wrong kind of food is eaten, or the person catches cold or has another disease, or he comes under emotional stress, the amount of insulin he is taking does not balance with the added bodily needs.

Stress—physical or emotional—increases the insulin requirements, and unfortunately emotional stress is frequently accompanied by an increase in food intake, thus increasing the gap between the amount of insulin provided and the need for it. Among rebellious adolescents especially, but in disturbed persons of any age or in persons subject to especially difficult problems, stress often creates medical crises. Their recurrence can be prevented only by social or psychiatric measures.

Signs of approaching coma are weariness, increased thirst, frequency and increased amount of urination, malaise, and vomiting. When these occur, the doctor should be called immediately or the person taken to the nearest hospital emergency room.

Another important factor which upsets control is unusual exercise. The exercise burns off food faster, so that the accustomed amount of insulin becomes excessive. Instead of going into acidosis or coma, he goes into insulin shock.

Signs of approaching shock are nervousness, apprehension, and sweating. There is often no warning, and the person loses consciousness suddenly. Fruit juice or sugar will ward off impending shock. Loss of consciousness requires emergency medical treatment.

The difficulty of staying in exact balance at all times can readily be seen. Some cases of diabetes are much more difficult to control than others, merely from an organic stand-point. Diabetes characterized by sudden fluctuation in blood sugar level is called *brittle* or *labile diabetes*. Persons whose occupations or recreation introduce irregular exercise, or children who are likely to exercise violently at unpredicta-ble times, find it hard to fit insulin requirements with metabolism. Irregularity in food intake upsets balance. The diabetic not only must remain within the general dietary restrictions but eat the same amount for each of the three meals every day as was prescribed when the insulin dosage was prescribed. If he eats less, or more, or distributes the food intake differently, he may have a serious crisis.

The insulin, the food, and the exercise must match. The personality and living habits of the individual must be taken into account when the treatment is being worked out by the doctor. These facts mean that: the individual treat-ment plan must be custom made by the physician, the per-son must stick with the plan faithfully, and if any untoward event (such as a cold) occurs he should see his doctor to work out a temporary change in plan.

One of the reasons for the individualization necessary is that there are three general types of insulin: (1) the fast-acting (regular and crystalline) insulin, which has a peak effect in about three to four hours; (2) the intermedi-ate-acting (NPH, lente and globin), which has maximal action in eight to ten hours; and slow-acting (protamine zinc, or PZI) which has a peak effect between twelve and twenty-four hours. In addition, mixtures are frequently used. The timing of the insulin and the kind given must be matched to the times when the food digestion most requires it. For these reasons *one type of insulin may never be substituted for another* without the doctor's orders and necessary changes in diet.

Self-administration of insulin requires conscientiousness

in sterilization of equipment and accuracy of dosage, sufficient eyesight to see the small markings on the syringe, and the capacity to mobilize one's will to stick a needle into oneself. Most persons can be taught to do these things. Occasionally social workers encounter clients who have severe psychological blockings against sticking themselves, but the common problems regarding insulin are those of poor eyesight and lack of understanding, money, and facilities.

Problems of insulin administration can be avoided among the group of diabetics who respond to recently developed insulin substitutes: medications taken by mouth. These oral medications (Orinase and Diabinese) are most often found useful for middle-aged persons who have not had diabetes for long. The continuous research and refinement in drugs make possible a wider application as time passes. The current use of oral insulin substitutes should therefore be investigated by workers who have clients with problems involving insulin administration.

The diabetic diet ranges in difficulty from the weighed diet, in which every mouthful must have first been weighed on a scale, to the so-called free diet. The latter is not prescribed by most physicians, although it is used as a compromise by some physicians with difficult patients, especially children and adolescents. It is not completely unrestricted, but does not purport to achieve the control of the usual standard diet.

In recent years most patients have been placed on a diet computed according to exchanges of food values (Exchange System) and by standard household measures instead of by grams. Food values are described on lists, and the individual may substitute one food for another of the same value. Although the Exchange System makes diet preparations much simpler than before, it still requires unusual knowledge of food values and the intellectual and emotional capacity necessary for self-denial and regulation.

In many cases the individual tailoring of food, insulin, and personality into a treatment plan should be done in a hospital. Trial and error are used in arriving at the kind and amount of insulin to give; food intake should be absolutely controlled during the experimental period; the urine must be collected and tested at frequent intervals. The patient must be taught how to administer his insulin, how to test his urine, how to compute the diet, and how to care for his feet so as to avoid the little irritations that might develop into gangrene.

During hospitalization the foundation is laid for the success or failure of the patient's continuing diabetic regime at home. If his learning experience has been successful, and if when he gets home neither economic, dietary, family, occupational, nor emotional problems interfere, he can begin the daily and lifelong attention to balancing his food intake, insulin activities, care of extremities, and maintenance of good physical resistance against infection. He will need to return regularly to the clinic or his private doctor for continued supervision.

COMPLICATIONS

The permanent complications which develop relate to the effect of diabetes on the blood vessels. The relationship of the disease to arteriosclerosis seems not to be completely understood or agreed upon. However, arteriosclerosis is a frequent accompaniment of diabetes, and its effects are speeded up by lack of control.

The effects of arteriosclerosis in the legs include poor circulation, which makes the danger of gangrene serious unless there is meticulous attention to care of the feet. The carbuncles and boils to which diabetics are subject are serious because of the difficulty of management when poor circulation exists.

An eye condition (*retinitis*), which may develop in diabetics with or without high blood pressure is called *diabetic retinopathy*. Permanent blindness results unless the diabetic condition is improved in time. The poor vision of many elderly and some young diabetics complicates management of self-administration of insulin, food preparation, and urine testing.

Diabetic neuropathy (nerve involvement), frequently affecting the extremities or the bladder, is another disabling complication of poorly controlled or advancing diabetes and, because of the pain, constitutes a handicap to employment and self-care. Like retinitis, it is an indication of a poor general condition and prognosis.

Heart trouble (specifically, coronary insufficiency) is one of the most formidable vascular complications, because of the danger of a heart attack or progressively severe cardiac limitations (described in chapter xi).

Tuberculosis and toxic goiter are two diseases sometimes found in association with diabetes. If either one exists, there is a mutually adverse effect between it and the diabetic condition. Thus these diseases should be considered among the complications of diabetes.

Implications for Public Assistance

As in dealing with any sick person, the public assistance worker needs first to find out from the client's physician what the medical situation dictates in regard to social planning. Mild diabetes in an older person, necessitating only minor adjustments, is a different matter from uncontrolled diabetes with complications, or any diabetes in a younger person.

QUESTIONS TO ASK THE PHYSICIAN

Is the diabetes mild, moderately severe, or severe? Is it responding well, or is it difficult to control? Have complications developed indicating permanent disability? If so, what are they and how limiting are they? What kind of diet is the client on—a weighed diet, standard diabetic diet, or free diet? Is insulin necessary? If so, is the client on long-lasting or short-acting insulin? How many daily injections must he give himself and at what times of day? Must he see a chiropodist regularly? How often does he need to attend clinic or come to the doctor's office? What special problems, if any, has the client manifested thus far?

Normally, we expect to concern ourselves with the client's needs in seven major areas: medical treatment, food, insulin, occupation, facilities for care of feet, complicating conditions or other diseases, and emotional stress.

INDIVIDUALIZATION OF TREATMENT

Except where mild diabetes occurs in an overweight adult and is controlled by a reducing diet alone, the amount of time and thought required for a tailor-made treatment plan is often not available in a county hospital clinic or a busy practitioner's office. In these circumstances the client can be expected to have difficulty staying in control. Many alert patients and families can be counted on to ask questions of the doctor, secure literature, and keep working until they find a satisfactory regime. However, in other circumstances the caseworker must take the initiative in calling a client's need to the attention of the hospital or physician. The worker may need to make sure that the client is seen by the dietitian, if food problems have not been satisfactorily worked out, or (with the concurrence of the doctor) secure the help of the public health department nutritionist or nurse.

INSULIN

When insulin administration poses a social or emotional problem, the worker should discuss the client's difficulty with the physician. In some instances he may be able to prescribe a longer-lasting insulin, which will make fewer injections necessary, or even one of the oral substitutes. It should be remembered that if the insulin is changed diet alterations will also have to be made. The worker may need to help the client return to the physician's office or clinic for the new instructions.

Some clients, especially young persons or those with emotional problems, find it impossible to inject themselves in front of other people: crowding and lack of privacy in the home may complicate matters. In these cases modification of living arrangements may be necessary to permit privacy. Provisions for sterilization of needles require minimum household equipment, but even this constitutes a problem under some marginal living plans. Urine testing can offer similar problems. Where failing eyesight causes difficulty to the client in reading the small gradations on the syringe, special syringes can be secured through resources known to those who work with the blind, or it may be possible to arrange for a relative, neighbor, or nurse to give the injections.

Storage of insulin requires refrigeration, although the open bottle does not have to be so kept. The distance the client lives from the source of insulin supply will influence whether or not he needs to keep several bottles on hand.

FOOD

The diabetic on a reducing diet will be hungry and under special temptation, but the diabetic person receiving insulin should be permitted enough food to keep from being hungry. The craving for forbidden sweets can be reduced to a certain extent through use of saccharin. Ordinarily, however, the rest of the family should try to make some sacrifices so as to reduce the temptation to the diabetic member.

Because the diabetic's food prescriptions call for unsweetened vegetables and fruits, ordinary canned food cannot be used. Home canning of unsweetened fruit is a substantial money-saver, if the agency and the recipient can devise means to utilize the food budget in a way which permits canning when fruit is available in the summer and fall.

Frozen vegetables and diabetic-pack canned fruit and fresh fruit raise the cost of the food budget. Low-cost meat is frequently high-fat, which is unsuitable.

Satisfying hunger on only lean meat, fruit, and vegetables is obviously expensive, but the diabetic cannot rely on the usual low-cost carbohydrates with which to meet his requirements. The rigidity of the diet, which prevents taking advantage of sales and necessitates more shopping and transportation, must also be considered. Diabetics cannot eat casserole dishes and mixtures unless each item that goes into them has been computed as part of the Exchange System and subtracted from the amounts allowed. This fact not only complicates usual low-income family cooking but raises the total cost.

Homemakers should be encouraged to take advantage of any food clinics where they can learn recipes and menus and share experiences with others who have similar cooking problems. This sometimes necessitates additional transportation or provision for babysitting.

Food is important in much of the recreation and social life in our culture. From school children's after-school or dating occasions to family gatherings and old persons' get-togethers, something good to eat (unfortunately often carbohydrates) is an important element. Then too, food has come to symbolize giving and receiving, and is frequently used as a reward to oneself or others.

Consequently the diabetic may either disregard his diet or feel deprived, abnormal, and lonely unless careful and considerate planning has gone into the social affairs he attends. The thoughtful homemaker can provide desserts for the diabetic by substituting items which he can have for those he cannot have. By using the Exchange System, he can go without a meal and eat an exchange at a party, but he must know how to do this and how to rearrange insulin dosage accordingly. He must also have the will power necessary.

The dietitian is an important resource where one is available through the county hospital clinic or the health department. In recent years some dietetic training courses have included an orientation in social factors in working with patients. Dietitians who have had experience in working with low-income groups have become accustomed to dealing with individuals who are not well prepared to master the complex subject of food components and values.

However, if the dietitian is not aware of a hiatus between her explanations and the client's capacity for understanding, it often helps for the worker to interpret the special needs of the client to her. In especially difficult cases, such as those of adolescents or individuals with cultural food problems, conferences can often be arranged which will enable the dietitian to be of maximum assistance to the client. Hospitals and physicians frequently recommend that patients buy a copy of Joslin's *Diabetic Manual*. Literate people of average intelligence find this standard text for lay persons an invaluable guide. It should be provided where either the budget or a private resource makes the book possible.

FOOT CARE

Important items for the diabetic include: well-fitting shoes with good soles, enough hose so that he will not need to wear any with holes or large darns, and living arrangements which enable him to wash his feet once a day. Any small irritation can result in a lesion that may eventually become gangrenous. The clothing allowance or extra private resources should be examined with this in mind.

A monthly visit to a chiropodist is often recommended by the physician; provision needs to be made for transportation and the necessary chiropody. It is considered dangerous for the diabetic to attempt his own foot care because of the hazard of cutting too deeply or of not giving adequate care to corns and calluses.

OCCUPATION

Two factors need to be taken into account in satisfactory employment, the first being to ascertain that the job does not entail an unpredictable amount of exertion. As has been pointed out, food and insulin requirements are predicted on a certain amount of exertion, and undue exercise may create insulin shock. Work which requires sudden bursts of energy—such as truck driving, with occasional loading of various heavy boxes—is considered unsuitable unless the client is well trained in management of his diabetes and knows how much extra sugar to ingest at the time of the unusual exercise. Airbons, lozenges, or orange juice are customarily used to prevent the adverse effects of unusual exercise. If a homemaker must perform certain heavy tasks at irregular intervals, such as scrubbing or doing hand laundry, she should discuss this matter with the physician in order to learn how to regulate food and insulin intake accordingly.

Lunch for the employed person may create difficulties. The individual who is on rapid-acting, short-lasting insulin may find it difficult to administer an injection during the lunch hour. If this is a problem it should be discussed with the doctor in order to learn whether the insulin prescription can and should be changed. The diabetic will usually need to carry his lunch if his work is in an industrial center where the eating facilities are confined to small enterprises with a limited choice of food, largely carbohydrate and fat-filled protein, such as hamburgers and pie.

COMPLICATING DISEASES

Diabetic neuropathy, resulting in painful legs and weakness, and diabetic retinopathy, resulting in poor vision, often create employment problems which may be difficult to evaluate. Because neuropathy is subjective and the pain not measurable, the physician may not be able to document unemployability in early cases. When the diabetic complains of being unable to work because of problems in his legs and feet, he should not be considered a hypochondriac even if the medical report indicates no objective signs. If the neuropathy becomes so severe that the skin ulcerates, the client will need close medical supervision, with assistance from the public health or visiting nurse if at all possible.

Vision is subject to changes in the diabetic whose blood-sugar levels vary. He may experience severe blurring without any actual pathology. If pathology exists, he may become temporarily improved with better attention to his underlying condition. However, major damage to the vessels in the eyes of the poorly controlled diabetic cannot be undone, and may usually be expected to progress slowly to blindness as his arteriosclerosis progresses with age. When the diabetic's eyesight is badly impaired, one of his first needs will be help in the administration of insulin, in order to avoid a vicious circle of poor vision and poor control.

The client who has tuberculosis and diabetes may be regarded as having a severe medical problem warranting special attention to the control of both diseases. Nutrition requires careful planning. The things that can be done to alleviate insecurity and emotional stress are important, as are good living conditions. Prevention of reactivation of tuberculosis, once it has been healed, also requires attention as to the kind of work the client may wish to return to, in order to make certain that it is suitable from the standpoint of the diabetes and the tuberculosis.

Surgery (including dental), pregnancy, and intermittent infections, offer temporary hazards unless medical management is thoughtful and the client willing and able to carry out the recommendations. Pregnancies need to be very closely supervised. Deliveries are ordinarily performed early by Caesarean section, because diabetic babies are large and subject to greater mortality than those of physically normal mothers. Common colds become a hazard if the diabetic has inadequate clothing for warmth and if the household is crowded.

EMOTIONAL STRESS

For many years it has been established that even animals excrete sugar in the urine when enraged or fearful, and that a rise in blood sugar occurs also in human beings. Because of the adverse effect of emotional stress upon the diabetic, the best efforts at medical control may fail if the client is chronically disturbed, resentful, or anxious. Coma is a recurring danger, especially when emotional upset causes the person rebelliously to disregard his diet or refuse to give himself the insulin he needs.

An understanding of the person is the basis for action. When the social study shows that the client is a seriously maladjusted person, efforts should be made in coöperation with the doctor to secure psychiatric help. However, if it seems that the individual has environmental, familial, economic, or occupational reasons to be disturbed, the casework resources of the agency and community can be tapped to alleviate the causes of the disturbed reactions.

Frequently, alleviation rather than cure of emotional stress is all that can be hoped for, but this is a worth-while goal and not impossible to achieve. The client's relationship with the agency can be made as constructive as possible through avoidance of conflict, reduction of insecurity in budget matters, a stable and helpful relationship with the worker, and use of all possible community resources. Keeping in touch with the doctor, so that he can be made aware of the client's social situation and can advise both the client and the worker from a medical standpoint, is helpful in coördinating medical-social treatment.

TERMS FREQUENTLY USED IN MEDICAL REPORTS

Acetone. A colorless liquid having a pleasant odor.

Acidosis. Technically a lowered blood bicarbonate; used to describe an abnormal condition in a diabetic which leads to coma and death if not corrected quickly.

Benedict's solution. A solution used in testing for sugar in the urine.

Brittle (or labile) diabetes. A form of diabetes in which levels of blood sugar change rapidly and are highly sensitive to insulin.

Clinitest. Test used for sugar in the urine.

Diuresis. Increased secretion of urine.

Exchange System. A method of diet computation. An "exchange" is the specific number of grams of fat, carbohydrate, protein, and calories to be found in a specified amount of food used as a basic unit in the Exchange System.

Furuncle. A boil.

Glucose tolerance test. A blood test used for detection of diabetes when diagnosis is uncertain.

Glycogen. The chief form of carbohydrate as stored in the body.

Glycosuria. The presence of an abnormal amount of sugar in the urine.

Hyperglycemia. A higher than normal concentration of sugar in the blood.

Hypoglycemia. A lower than normal concentration of sugar in the blood.

Insulin resistance. A condition in which large doses of insulin do not achieve the expected control.

Ketonuria. The presence of ketones in the urine.

Ketosis. An excessive production of ketones in the blood which causes coma.

Neuropathy. A disorder of the nervous system presenting bizarre symptoms of altered sensation, pain, muscle function, and function of gastrointestinal and urinary tracts.

Polydipsia. Excessive thirst.

Polyuria. The passage of abnormally large amount of urine.

Pruritis. Intense itching.

Pruritis vulvae. Intense itching of the external genitals of the female.

Retinitis. Inflammation of the retina.

Retinopathy. Any noninflammatory disease of the retina.

Uremia. A toxic condition caused by suppression or insufficient secretion of urine in which urinary constituents remain in the blood.

CHAPTER V

Tuberculosis

IN THE GENERAL REJOICING about the dramatic reduction in mortality from tuberculosis, danger exists that social workers may not appreciate what a vast problem it remains in public assistance caseloads. Not only is the disease still common among assistance recipients, but it carries particularly grave social responsibilities.

Contrary to the general impression, the number of newly reported cases each year remains almost as great as ever. Further, tuberculosis is not, as some seem to think, a disease now confined to skid road inhabitants. Half the new cases occur in persons less than 43 years of age, and about half the total group are married. The disease is particularly dangerous to young children, adolescents, and women who have just delivered a child.

Family and child welfare workers share with those who work with the aged and disabled a need to be informed about a disease which is infectious, which can be fatal (especially in children), and which always causes major social disturbance when it attacks. Curiously enough, at a time when improved medical treatment has reduced the extent of social damage, through reducing the length and seriousness of the illness, the social worker's participation in treatment is more important than ever.

Half the persons with tuberculosis are said to be at home. They have either been sent to a sanatorium and have left against advice or have been sent home after a brief institutional stay to carry out drug treatment at home. Studies have shown that a distressingly large number have far-advanced disease, and receive only nominal medical attention or none at all.

Racial groups have varying degrees of natural resistance to tuberculosis, just as families and individuals do. Persons with tuberculosis who come from groups with poor resistance are especially vulnerable to the disease, thus needing special concern and attention. Negroes, American Indians, and Chinese are among them. The thin-skinned, titian-haired groups, such as the Irish, are also thought to have low resistance to tuberculosis.

Tuberculosis is a disease which is frequently associated with lowered bodily resistance, poor nutrition, overcrowding, and poor hygienic conditions. Thus it can readily be seen that both prevention and treatment often require the tools of the social worker; the budgeting and other services she provides have a direct relation to the control of the recipient's disease.

General Medical Base for Social Planning

THE LUNGS

Tuberculosis can occur in almost any part of the body, particularly the lungs, bones, glands and kidneys. Because it is most frequently a disease of the lungs, the discussion here is confined to this form of the disease—*pulmonary tuberculosis*.

It is helpful to visualize the lungs and how they are attacked. If one imagines an inverted tree, the trunk beginning in the throat, and the branches (bronchi) and twigs (bronchioles) extending into the chest cavity, one gets a fairly accurate picture of the literally named bronchial tree. Put thousands of tiny leaves on the tree, and one has the air sacs (alveoli) in which are exchanged the oxygen from breathing and the carbon dioxide from the blood.

The trees and its leaves are paired into two lungs, one of which has three lobes and the other two lobes, and are surrounded by a membrane called the pleura. The air sacs are intertwined with numerous tiny blood vessels and capillaries. When a person breathes, bellows-fashion, the sacs fill and the walls of the capillaries are so fine that they permit the pure air to enter the blood and the impure gases to be exhaled. Thus the lungs perform one of their main functions: purifying the blood.

ONSET AND COURSE

Tuberculosis is contracted by inhaling *tubercle bacilli* exhaled by someone in an infectious stage of the disease. A person whose resistance is high can throw off a few bacilli, so there is little danger to a person, such as a social worker if she is only occasionally exposed. On the other hand, in repeated contact with someone who has active disease, the amount of infection may be so overwhelming that even though the individual's body resistance is high he may not be able to ward off the infection and may develop tuberculosis within a few weeks or months. Of course this is more likely to occur if the individual is in a run-down condition. Then even a small number of organisms inhaled can cause disease.

When the bacilli burrow into the delicate air sacs, they multiply like moths in wool. Because of the inflammation and the sloughing-off process that they cause, holes or cavities result. When the infection spreads into blood vessels, hemorrhage (*hemoptysis*) results, which is not only a frightening (and sometimes fatal) experience but one which may do considerable damage by spreading the disease further into the lungs or causing pneumonia.

Tuberculosis has no symptoms other than laziness and fatigue at first, with later loss of weight, cough, slight temperature, and night sweats. Consequently, persons often do not know they have tuberculosis in the early stages, unless they have a small early hemorrhage which sends them to the doctor or the disease is discovered by a routine chest X ray. They may refuse to believe the diagnosis or to have treatment, because they are in no pain and feel so nearly normal.

Just how slowly or rapidly the disease may progress is a highly individual matter, depending upon the number of germs inhaled, the individual body condition and resistance, the race and age of the patient. In addition, other infections, hemorrhages, nutrition, and quality of medical care are important factors.

Young children and adolescents may develop acute and serious forms of tuberculosis, which have often run rapidly fatal courses in the past. Fortunately, improved diagnostic techniques and modern drugs can control this acute phase of the disease so that today most children and young persons can be saved, even from severe infections. The period immediately after delivery of a child is a highly critical one for the tuberculous woman.

Just as the disease may advance slowly with no outward warning, the healing process is also slow. The body's natural defenses attempt to wall off the bacilli with a cheeselike substance which grows out of the fibrous scars and eventually calcifies and permanently walls off the bacilli. However, the hardening process is extremely slow, so that the protective wall can be easily broken down at any time within several years.

Even after this calcification is complete, the dormant tubercle bacilli may break through many years later and cause the individual to have a reactivation. Large cavities are always difficult to heal completely by natural process, and break down more readily than do small ones. This accounts for the danger of relapse in tuberculosis. This characteristic of the disease is one of the most damaging to the personality and work capacity of the patient: he always has a sword of Damocles hanging over his head.

The worker in the aid-to-disabled program is especially concerned with the scarring process, because the healing of extensive disease results in widespread substitution of inelastic fibrous and calcified areas for lung tissue. This means that the individual cannot get enough air to perform normal activities, and he is *dyspneic* or short of breath on slight exertion. The same results may occur if some parts of the lung have been removed by surgery and other parts are scarred from battles with the bacilli. A severe pulmonary cripple is, of course, permanently disabled. (See Chapter vi for discussion of this condition.)

TREATMENT

There are three kinds of treatment, and usually two or more are applied at the same time. The first and most important is promoting the body's own natural defenses, which is accomplished by rest and good nutrition. No matter what else is done, the individual cannot become well unless his bodily defenses work effectively; although the new drugs keep the bacilli from multiplying, they do not kill the bacilli which are already there, nor can they replace lost tissue.

The drugs which have become such an important mainstay of treatment are especially effective in relatively fresh, spreading tuberculosis. The three predominant drugs are streptomycin and its derivatives and *I.N.H.* and *P.A.S.* Streptomycin has had some very unfortunate toxic effects, making people dizzy and sometimes permanently deaf. It is now used safely in smaller doses in combination with the other drugs.

P.A.S. may be irritating to the stomach, causing nausea and pain. The flexible, understanding doctor will work until he finds the effective combination of drugs which is neither unpleasant nor dangerous. However, it is not always to be assumed that the patient who is "uncoöperative" in taking his drugs is arbitrarily or capriciously so.

At present, drugs are usually prescribed for about two years after the beginning of treatment, but some patients must take them all their lives.

Pill taking would seem to be a simple treatment measure, easy for the patient to carry out. Many persons, however, do not continue with their medications, possibly because taking pills regularly seems so prosaic that its importance is not fully comprehended.

Radical lung surgery is the third prong of modern treatment. Before advanced techniques made removal or *resection* of lobes or a whole lung possible, collapse techniques were widely used to give the lung complete rest even from breathing. Air was injected by needle into the pleural cavity (*pneumothorax*) or into the abdomen (*pneumoperitoneum*), or a nerve was cut to force up the diaphragm. These techniques, no longer used to any extent, flattened the lung or a part of it.

Permanent collapse was also achieved by a major operation called *thoracoplasty* which involved removing the ribs. This operation is still used in some institutions in conjunction with lobe- or lung-removal but has generally been abandoned. It creates an unsightly deformity and is painful postoperatively.

Pulmonary resection (removing parts of lung tissue) is now the principal form of surgery and is not outwardly mutilating. *Lobectomy* (removal of one lobe) may be performed if this will cut out a big cavity or the most infected site; *pneumonectomy* (removal of a whole lung) may be necessary. Plastic balls may be put in to fill the space, or a *pleural flap* may be made, or thoracoplasty may be performed to keep the space left by removal of the lung from filling with fluid.

Although the mortality from pulmonary resection in good institutions is low, these operations are major indeed, both in terms of risk and in terms of postoperative pain and possibility of complications. Clients have every right to be fearful and to need all the support which their families and social workers can give them.

Implications for Public Assistance

QUESTIONS TO ASK THE DOCTOR

It is not enough to know that a client has tuberculosis. One must find out from the public health department or private doctor whether the client is infectious or not (sputum positive or negative); whether his disease is active or inactive; whether he needs treatment and, if so, what kind; how long he will need to be away if sanatorium care is recommended; what the prognosis is if the disease is still active; and, for those who have been discharged from the sanatorium, what the work tolerance is if any.

When the client has long-time tuberculosis and the worker suspects, from the client's general fatigability and shortness of breath, that he may be a "pulmonary cripple," she should ask specifically about reduced *vital capacity* (a measure of lung function) and what this implies about kinds of work, if any, that the client may be physically able to perform. If the client has been in a sanatorium which has a social service department, the worker should ascertain from the hospital social worker what kind of adjustment he made, and whether there are social problems the welfare department should be aware of.

EMOTIONAL RAMIFICATIONS

Persons with tuberculosis are likely to feel disgraced, even in this time of intellectual enlightenment, possibly because the disease is widely associated with poverty and poor living conditions. Although poverty may have had nothing to do with their disease, or although they may have been innocent victims of contagion, they find in the sanatorium a large number of persons from underprivileged groups and so they feel stigmatized.

Knowledge of having an infectious condition makes some persons feel unclean or like "Typhoid Mary." This feeling is aggravated by their having to wear masks, carefully to keep dishes and towels separate, expectorate into tissues that must be placed in paper bags and burned. Also, conscientious persons may feel guilty about the possibility of having infected others, especially their children, before they knew they had the disease. Neurotic fears may build up that they are being punished for something—a common reaction to catastrophe. Fear of tuberculosis is widespread.

Early case finding and brief (less than a year), effective treatment now make it possible for many patients, especially young ones, to get back into the stream of life without permanent damage to their relationships and personality. Those who have had serious disease will always have to put their health first, something that is obviously hard to do. Most will need to avoid prolonged exposure, hard physical labor, severe mental stress, late hours, and excesses of all kinds throughout their lives; they will also need to remain under some form of medical supervision, to make sure that they have not become active and infectious again. Further, they may find potential employers unwilling to hire them, and some co-workers ignorantly afraid of them.

Any major disease occurs not in a vacuum but in the midst of a welter of activities, worries, relationships, goals, and fears, entirely unrelated to the disease entity. The patient is first and foremost a person, with individual concerns and characteristics. These will affect the way in which he responds to the disease and to its treatment requirements.

Going to the sanatorium, for example, may be relatively welcome to a tired, embattled old man with no home; but it may be catastrophic to a young girl in love, or to the father of three children who has just built a new house, and bought furniture and a car on the installment plan. The person with many inner resources and an adaptable temperament may be able to adjust to the role of patient with relative ease. However, the proud, independent person or the individual who needs to cling hard to precarious independence may find it almost intolerable to put aside his own desires and do what the doctor and nurses tell him to do.

Some states have public health laws which force persons with active tuberculosis to go to a sanatorium and to remain there until they are no longer infectious. Such laws remove from the individual the need for a decision as to whether he will enter an institution, and may be almost a relief to those persons who are in conflict and cannot make up their minds to impose institutional restrictions upon themselves.

Any law which deprives an individual of his liberty is dangerous, and must be administered with great care. Extra effort needs to be made to be sure that the individual's feelings are understood and that his social needs are met. The social worker has an obligation to help him to the best of her ability, to take care of the affairs that may be troubling him. If the individual is angry that authority has been imposed upon him, it is helpful to give him an opportunity to "let off steam" and to express understanding in a nonjudging manner.

After having made the adjustment, at whatever price, to the treatment for tuberculosis some persons who have recovered are afraid to meet the competition of the outside world again. They have seen too many chronic invalids at the sanatorium; they have heard too many stories of disappointment or breakdown after normal activity; they may have watched others die or heard the groans of the postoperative. Long or repeated sanatorium stays are often so demoralizing that many do not recover normal initiative again.

SPECIAL HOUSING CONSIDERATIONS

The client with infectious disease should not remain in the home with small children or adolescents; if there is a child under three or an adolescent in the home, either the child or the client should be removed as quickly as possible— the client preferably to a treatment facility. Possible exceptions may occasionally exist if home environment, intelligence, and conscientiousness are far above average. However, the separation of a tuberculous person from young children is generally one of the most urgent of all social measures.

Bedclothing, including pillows and mattresses, is a continuing source of tubercle bacilli after the infectious client has been removed. Bedding should be aired in bright sun for three days or handled in accord with the instructions of the public health nurse or, if necessary, destroyed. Some mattresses and pillows may need to be destroyed and replaced. Private resources can usually be tapped for this purpose beyond the amounts permitted in the budget.

The client who returns from the sanatorium or who is awaiting sanatorium care, should have a bed of his own in a room of his own. Private sleeping arrangements are vital if he is infectious, and are desirable during the period his disease is active whether his sputum is positive or not. These arrangements can be made in a variety of ways. In some instances maximum use of the housing allowance in budgeting basic needs will suffice; in others, budgetary provision for special or extra needs will be necessary and feasible; in still others, private agency resources or help from relatives may be tapped.

Items especially needed will include a comfortable mattress and sufficient bedding for cleanliness and warmth and, if the client is infectious, separate towels, toilet articles, and enough dishes so that his can be kept separate. Where policy permits a family to retain a television they have started to buy, it is helpful in promoting rest and relaxation.

OTHER CHARACTERISTIC NEEDS

Good nutrition is a major requirement of the tuberculous client and of exposed family members; special diet allowances should be provided in the budget. The other family members should be on preventive, high-caloric, high-protein diets as long as necessary. Where a young adult client has had a thoracoplasty and is deformed, and especially where employment is a possibility, the need for especially designed clothing to make the deformity less noticeable may also need to be taken into account. If he is in bed at home, he will need extra pajamas and a robe and slippers.

Avoidance of stress is the companion piece to good nutrition in helping the client to get well or to stay well. Consequently, a continuing plan, which will provide him with some sense of security, is highly desirable. Checks should not be held up unless it is absolutely necessary. Those things that can be done to reduce the client's worries, such as enabling the spouse to visit him while he is in the sanatorium, take on great importance in treatment.

THE ALCOHOLIC

What to do about the alcoholic client who "drinks up his assistance check" is a difficult problem. Withholding the check, the means of his obtaining food, when this may create reactivation of his tuberculosis, is certainly false economy. Because case finding has been concentrated in recent years upon the jails and skid roads, a proportionately large number of tuberculous homeless men with personality problems have been identified. Many of these use alcohol to excess.

That alcoholism is a disease, not a moral problem, is generally conceded. We have passed beyond the day of the "you straighten up" approach. For a time, social workers and psychiatrists felt that alcoholism was a hopeless disease, but fortunately this feeling is passing too. Alcoholism is now considered to be an emotional illness due to a variety of causes, some of which respond to treatment and some of which do not.

In the tuberculosis sanatorium many alcoholics get along relatively well, if a personal interest is taken in them and they feel that someone cares. Their physical needs for food and shelter are met, and they are in a nontempting environment. However, if upon sanatorium discharge skid road is the only place of refuge, relapse into alcoholism and reactivation of tuberculosis seem almost inevitable. Dr. Dan Morse, a tuberculosis sanatorium director in Illinois, has put it well: "One of the worst obstacles to preventing reactivation in an alcoholic who has succeeded in bringing his tuberculosis under control is the bad environment in which he is likely to find himself after release from a sanatorium. Everything seems to act as an incentive toward renewed drinking: idleness and inactivity brought about by convalescence, the low economic situation, domestic troubles, misdirection of friends and family, and the desire for temporary relief from worries." *

For people who are destitute and homeless, provision must first be made for shelter, food, and clothing. Relieving insecurity about fundamental physical needs and providing a decent environment are the first steps in the helping process. A sustained, supportive interest which provides human warmth and concern, but is still realistic about the problem and expects the client to do his part, is the other half of the client's fundamental need.

Valiant attempts to help the tuberculous alcoholic are being made in a number of communities. For example, Sacramento, California, is achieving substantial success as a result of dedicated pooled effort by the county welfare department, the tuberculosis control officer, public health nurses, the tuberculosis association, the Alcoholic Rehabilitation Clinic, Alcoholics Anonymous, and a private individual with unusual compassion and capacity. Small caseloads, a carefully defined approach, clear-cut rules,

---

* Dan Morse, M.D., "Alcohol and Tuberculosis," *NTA Bulletin,* Nov., 1956.

group living with planned work and recreational activity, group and individual psychotherapy for those who can use it, a wholesome environment, with the important addition of personal interest in the individuals—seem to constitute the responsible combination.

In the Sacramento experiment, several county welfare department plans exist to fit the needs and characteristics of different individuals. They are set up to provide assistance to alcoholics who want to rehabilitate themselves. Services and funds are concentrated on those clients who can accept some limitations and who are motivated to coöperate in staying sober and getting well. Vendor payments are used for meals, grocery orders, shelter, or for congregate living.

Two county welfare department workers specialize in carrying responsibility for services to tuberculosis patients. They work closely with the clients, the health department personnel, the manager of the congregate facilities, and the psychiatrist and social worker of the Alcoholic Rehabilitation Clinic. A rudimentary but pleasant "camp" in a peaceful country setting—Altua Village—and a board-and-care home in the city are operated by the unusual manager. Maintenance work is required from each client for no more than four hours a day, but various volunteer work projects further occupy those who are interested.

The county welfare department deserves great credit for the work which is going forward, but James Boock, Chief of the General Assistance–Aid to Disabled Division, modestly ascribes the values gained to all the various organizations and persons who have combined their efforts: "All . . . rolled up their sleeves and really went to work on this difficult community problem. We have been blessed with some very favorable results because of the dedicated effort on the part of so many individuals and agencies." *

---

* Unpublished material, James Boock, Supervisor, Sacramento Department of Public Welfare, March 18, 1960.

EMPLOYMENT

Suitable employment for persons with healed tuberculosis is not so hard to find as it was before drug treatment. Most individuals are not infectious as long as they were formerly. Some physicians allow patients who had minimal disease and who are well healed to return to hard physical labor. Less discrimination among employers is encountered against the person whose tuberculosis is healed and who remains under medical supervision. The vocational rehabilitation agencies accept many persons with healed tuberculosis who need job counseling, retraining, and assistance in job placement.

In spite of these assets, employment remains a serious problem for the many whose age, lack of education, and personality factors, combined with the handicap of tuberculosis, reduce to a minimum the number of available suitable jobs. Deterioration in capacity and motivation occurs during the waiting period unless Herculean efforts are made to substitute for the social values of employment in other ways. Sheltered workshop employment, group recreational activities, pursuit of hobbies, and participation in household or family responsibilities are some of the means by which the person can retain the morale necessary to keep open the possibility of employment. Thus, a long-continuing joint effort on the part of recipient, social worker, vocational counselor, and physician is often necessary before the recipient with tuberculosis is "rehabilitated." Many former patients in the older age group will never return to the satisfaction of self-support, but it is incumbent upon us to try wholeheartedly to reduce this number in every way we can.

TERMS FREQUENTLY USED IN MEDICAL REPORTS *

Acid-fast. A laboratory method referring to characteristics of the tubercle bacillus; thus synonymous with tubercle bacillus in common parlance.

Active, activity. Describes disease that is not healed. Ongoing disease process.

AMA (AWOL). Patient left hospital "Against Medical Advice" (Away Without Leave); also described as "Irregular Discharge."

Arrested TB. Disease process appears to have been stopped (the term "inactive" is now used instead of "arrested").

BCG. Vaccine against tuberculosis.

Bilateral. Describes disease in both lungs.

Calcification. Late healing process wherein lime salts are deposited in the tissues.

Cavity. A hole produced in the lung by certain diseases.

Chemotherapy. Treatment by medicine or drugs.

Communicable. Infectious, contagious. Transmissible from person to person.

Contact. A person who has been in continued and/or close touch with a patient with active tuberculosis.

Culture. Mass of micro-organisms growing in certain media in a laboratory; used for test purposes.

Drug resistance. Condition in which the strain of tubercles present is one not affected by the drugs in use to combat tuberculosis.

Empyema. Accumulation of pus in the space between lung and chest wall because of infection.

Far advanced. Official classification for tuberculosis in an advanced stage to signify the extent of the lung tissue involved.

Gastric lavage. A method of obtaining a sample of sputum from the gastric contents by means of a tube passed into the stomach.

---

* From glossary prepared by Subcommittee on Public Assistance of the California Tuberculosis Association.

Hemoptysis. Spitting up blood; a blood-stained sputum.

Infectious. Contagious, communicable; describes disease caused by parasites or germs.

I.N.H. (Isoniazid). One of the drugs used to treat tuberculosis.

Lesion. A wound in body tissue.

Lobectomy. Surgical removal of a lobe of the lung.

Mantoux test. Injection of tuberculin into the skin to test for the presence of tuberculous infection. A positive reaction does not necessarily indicate that the person has active tuberculosis.

Miliary. An acute form of tuberculosis in which the disease is spread, by way of the blood stream, through the body.

Minifilm. Small X-ray pictures.

Minimal. Official classification of tuberculosis in which lesions are small and only a small part of the lungs is affected.

Moderately advanced. Official classification of the disease stage between minimal and far advanced.

Nonpulmonary. Describes tuberculosis of parts of the body other than the lungs.

P.A.S. (Paraminosalicylic acid). One of the drugs used in treatment of tuberculosis, usually combined with other drugs.

Patch test. Test of skin sensitivity to tuberculin, administered by means of a plaster or patch. Not as reliable as a Mantoux test.

Phrenic nerve. Nerve controlling the diaphragm. In treatment this nerve may be surgically "crushed" in order to produce a temporary paralysis, or it may be removed by *phrenectomy*.

Pneumonectomy. Surgical removal of one lung.

Pneumoperitoneum (PNP). Injection of air into the abdominal cavity to collapse the lung.

Pneumothorax. Injection of air into the pleural cavity in order to produce partial collapse of the lung.

Positive. Describes condition when tubercle bacilli are present.

Primary tuberculosis. The disease process which results from initial infection with tubercle bacilli.

Pulmonary. Referring to the lung.

Reactivation. Condition when inactive tuberculosis has again
become active.

Resection. Surgical removal of part of the lung.

Streptomycin (strep). Drug used in treatment of tuberculosis
(by injection).

Thoracic. Of the chest wall or rib cage.

Thoracentesis. Surgical puncture or tapping of the chest wall.

Thoracoplasty. Surgical removal of ribs to produce collapse of
the lung.

Tubercle bacillus. Germ which causes tuberculosis.

Tuberculin. Substance used in skin sensitivity tests to determine
the presence of tuberculous infection.

Unilateral. Onesided; describes disease in one lung.

Vital capacity. A test of the amount of air the lungs can expel,
frequently used to determine how adequately the lungs function.

CHAPTER VI

The Pulmonary Cripple

THE PULMONARY OR RESPIRATORY CRIPPLE is handicapped by shortness of breath. Various chest conditions may cause this type of crippling, including the end results of old tuberculosis, radical lung surgery, bronchiectasis, silicosis, and other similar diseases. However, the major causes of pulmonary crippling are long-standing chronic bronchial asthma and emphysema. Consequently this chapter discusses these conditions. From a practical standpoint, what is said about the effects of emphysema can also be applied to other far-advanced chronic chest conditions.

Asthma and emphysema are related to each other in that asthma often leads to emphysema, and both are characterized by difficulty in breathing. We lack an accurate picture of the number of pulmonary cripples who have advanced stages of these conditions, but we know that they exist in increasing numbers and that their progressive disability leads to inability to work and therefore often to financial dependence.

Asthma occurs in both sexes and in any age group, but emphysema is predominantly a disease occurring after the age of fifty. Most sufferers who come to attention are men, perhaps because the economic consequences of shortness of breath are more marked in them. Neither emphysema nor chronic asthma is curable, although some asthmatic children recover spontaneously.

General Medical Base for Social Planning

ONSET AND COURSE

The causes of asthma and emphysema are manifold. Allergies, respiratory infections, and emotional disturbances are considered causative in asthma. Approximately half the asthma cases are said to be caused by extrinsic or outside factors such as pollens or dust, and the other half by intrinsic factors or those inside the person such as respiratory infection. The asthmatic attack itself is the result of intermittent spasms of the bronchial tubes and excessive mucus in the bronchi. Some patients live normally between attacks, but others wheeze continually and are more or less constantly incapacitated. A patient who goes into one attack after another, with the bronchi constantly in acute spasm, is said to be in *status asthmaticus*. This is an emergency condition which requires close medical attendance.

During a spasm, air that has been inhaled cannot be exhaled; the result is an overextension of the air sacs of the lungs. This hyperinflation subsides when the spasm ends, but if it happens often enough and long enough the lungs become permanently dilated and lose their elasticity. The fine circulatory structure of the lungs is damaged, and the heart has difficulty pumping blood through the vessels. The air sacs break down, and the patient cannot expel air efficiently. Tenacious sputum forms which is hard to cough up. Body chemistry is distorted. The impure air or carbon dioxide cannot be exhaled, and not enough oxygen can be inhaled. Such a person is said to be *emphysematous,* or he has developed *chronic generalized obstructive pulmonary emphysema.*

Chronic asthma is not the only cause of emphysema. Air pollution in big cities or in certain occupations, smoking, repeated respiratory infections, and simply the process of aging with the accompanying changes in chest contour and lung tissue—all play a part. Usually the individual is not aware of the gradual changes in his lungs until he has pneumonia or some acute respiratory illness, after which his emphysema becomes much worse.

He becomes so short of breath that he cannot carry on the ordinary activities of daily life without great effort and fatigue. Exertion sends him into bouts of coughing. He is troubled with tenacious sputum which he tries to clear from his throat. At this advanced stage there is no way that medical science can prevent the relentless progression of his disease. The client will become severely incapacitated and die within a few years from heart failure or from insufficient oxygen in the blood.

DIAGNOSIS

The manner in which the doctor makes a diagnosis is of some interest in providing clues as to the significance of medical reports. He orders chest X rays and fluoroscopy to see areas of fibrosis or scarring; secures blood studies to determine the chemical composition and whether too many red blood cells are being manufactured to compensate for lack of oxygen; listens to the chest for the noises, *rales;* measures the chest upon inspiration, and notes the almost nonexistent differential caused by the state of permanent expansion of the chest walls; watches for evidence of *barrel chest;* checks for blueness of the nail beds and skin to ascertain whether *cyanosis* has already developed; checks and records any signs of heart impairment, such as swelling of the ankles, murmurs, fast pulse, irregularity, to see whether the strain has begun to cause *cor pulmonale* (right-sided heart failure).

TREATMENT

Treatment of asthma attempts to remove the precipitating factors and relieve the symptoms; treatment of emphysema is designed to relieve the severe distress of clients with these diseases. Many social adjustments may be necessary for the asthmatic whose illness is caused chiefly by allergy to some factor in the occupation, housing, or diet.

Since fear or anxiety is thought to be both a cause and a result of asthma, security, calm, and optimism are important in treatment. In addition, effort must be made to overcome any existing allergic factors, which may involve such practical matters as special diet, plastic mattress and pillow covers, replacement of wool clothing and blankets with cotton or synthetic materials, the use of plastic or air-foam textiles in furnishings, and a dust-free environment without cats, dogs, or birds.

Asthma caused by respiratory infections is treated with antibiotics and other medications. A strict no-smoking regime is advised for all asthmatics and emphysematous patients. Extra rest and maximum diet are also considered essential for all with these conditions.

In both asthma and emphysema, medications are urgently required: to liquefy sputum, relieve bronchial spasm, control or mitigate infections, and attempt to control heart failure if it is present. The client may often need a nebulizer or hand spray to administer his own medicine for spasm.

He must have immediate access to a physician or to a hospital in a crisis.

Oxygen administration, one of the important features of treatment, may be carried out by an oxygen tent or mask, with a tank at the bedside for temporary relief of symptoms. Administration of oxygen by a special machine (Bennet Valve) has brought temporary relief to many emphysema patients, even though the measurable or laboratory improvement is often negligible. Such treatments are called Intermittent Positive Pressure Breathing (IPPB) and are usually administered in a clinic or a physician's office.

In an attempt to avoid hospitalization or to discharge hospital patients home who have severe emphysema and whose active hospital treatment consists primarily of IPPB treatments, some physicians will suggest that patients rent or buy a machine for home use. The social worker should discuss a recommendation of this kind with the agency medical consultant before participating in such a plan, because some doctors believe severe dangers exist in self-administration of oxygen with an IPPB machine. If the plan is worked out, provision should be made for adequate supervision.

"Emphysema belts" may be prescribed to hold the diaphragm in place as a mechanical aid in expelling air from the lung, although some authorities believe that they are of little benefit. Others think they are important for selected patients.

Combating weight loss is another urgent part of treatment. Loss of appetite and poor nutrition add to the patient's fatigue and debility, and make him more prone to infection.

EFFECTS OF THE DISEASE

The distress of acute attacks and of progressive shortness of breath (dyspnea) and increasing debility are the outstanding characteristics of asthma and emphysema. "Perhaps the most compelling of all human appetites is the need for air and probably no distress is so agonizing as that which results from the inability to breathe adequately." * Excessive fatigue, to the point where merely getting dressed is a chore and even talking is tiresome, is a usual symptom of advanced disease. There is usually progressive loss of weight and absence of appetite in the late stages of the disease, with despair and futility as concomitants.

Inability to sleep lying down adds to the fatigue and discomfort. In late stages of asthma and emphysema, the patient must prop himself up on more and more pillows as his condition progresses, and finally he has to try to sleep sitting in a chair. Treatment can often bring relief from symptoms for a time, to the extent that the individual can go back to work or can carry on some form of sedentary employment temporarily.

Implications for Public Assistance

The first need of the asthmatic or emphysematous recipient is good medical care, including the practical items which make medical treatment effective. Early attention can prevent or postpone the costly invalidism which otherwise will result.

Psychotherapy may be indicated for asthmatic individuals with serious personality problems. By the time the asthmatic has become middle-aged and/or emphysematous, it is often too late to help him change his emotional patterns of reacting to events and emotions. If psychiatric facilities are limited, it would seem sounder to use them for asth-

---

* Horton Corwin Hinshaw, M.D., and Henry L. Garland, M.B., B.Ch., *Diseases of the Chest* (Philadelphia: W. B. Saunders Co., 1956), p. 230.

matic children unless some exceptional circumstances exists.

The most realistic goal in most cases is social treatment designed to promote good medical care, a comfortable and dustfree environment when indicated, maximum security, and reduction of tensions, hardships, and physical exertion.

INDIVIDUALIZATION OF THE MEDICAL CONDITION

The recipient who has bronchial asthma and/or emphysema or some other chronic lung condition which creates pulmonary crippling needs, like other ill persons, an understanding of his particular medical problem (and, of course, his temperament and social situation, for the handicap cannot be treated separately from the individual who has the illness).

Is he an asthmatic, subject to unpredictable emergency attacks? If so, to what does the doctor ascribe the primary cause—pollens or dust or something from which the recipient could escape? Or is it a respiratory infection? Or does the basic problem seem to be fear and insecurity? If the patient does not have acute attacks, but rather is disabled by constant difficulty in getting his breath and by his fatigue and weakness, we know we have a different problem. In either case, what is most necessary from a practical standpoint? The answer to these questions must be obtained from the physician. If the recipient has not been told or has not understood what his treatment goals should be, then arrangements should be made for the doctor to talk with him.

SPECIAL NEEDS OF THE ASTHMATIC

Asthma that is allergic in nature may require major social adjustments. The farmer who is allergic to animal danders may have to give up farming and receive training through

VRS for a new occupation; the homeowner who is allergic to olive trees in his backyard may have to remove the trees or sell the property; the family or recipient may have to move to a different location free from the pollens or industrial smoke of the area.

Change of climate to avoid damp and cold is sometimes recommended. A medical recommendation to this effect should be discussed carefully with the physician, for a major move could bring more disadvantages than advantages. Loneliness, anxiety, and problems in securing housing and medical care must be taken into account.

Change of climate should not, however, be summarily dismissed as impractical for persons who happen to live in especially disadvantageous places. A move to another community, accompanied by the necessary detailed planning, may prove a humane and economical move. A trial period for the recipient before the whole family is uprooted is ideal, for the expected advantage may not materialize.

Practical planning with the asthmatic should take into account the unpredictable and emergency nature of acute attacks and the client's anxiety about them. He requires the security of knowing that he can have emergency care when he needs it, either at a hospital emergency room or from a private physician. The recipient should have a telephone, and transportation by automobile or taxi should be always accessible. The source of medical care should be satisfactory to the recipient, or, propelled by his fear, he will use money budgeted for other needs to secure care that he does believe adequate.

Medical care may be costly, including antibiotics prescribed to combat acute infection, medical supplies such as a nebulizer and syringe, tranquilizers to allay fear, and oxygen. If the clinic pharmacy does not stock the drugs which the doctor has prescribed or the recipient has found helpful, he will usually try to get them from a private drugstore.

In other words, the recipient whose health problem subjects him to emergencies may be in constant difficulty in regard to budget, borrowing funds for emergency taxis, or for food to last until the end of the month, or some new medicine, unless the worker plans ahead with him as to how his medical needs will be met. The recipient who is always upset will become worse physically—a vicious circle resulting.

Consequently, uncertainties over the assistance check should be reduced to a minimum, and basic and special-need items and community resources should be fully utilized. When a recipient spends money from his grant for emergency medical needs, the worker should arrange for reimbursement, whenever possible, to enable him to meet regularly budgeted needs for the remainder of the budget period. The agency's policy and provision for supplemental funds should be discussed with the recipient, so that he will know that he has to report emergencies and what to expect in the way of reimbursement.

HOUSING

One of the most important ways in which the asthmatic or emphysematous person can be helped is through attention to housing. If he is close to medical care, much expense can be avoided. If a dust-free environment has been advised by the physician, the recipient who does his own housekeeping should have more than one room. This makes possible a bedroom which can be stripped of dust catchers, the floor mopped daily, and the bed appropriately made up with plastic covers and cotton blankets; in other words a refuge from dust, an important health resource.

When the recipient is single, as is frequently true, the

effort of housekeeping should be kept in mind, because the pulmonary cripple is weak and frail and impeded by shortness of breath. First-floor housing is essential, especially if there is heart involvement.

A boarding house or nursing home offers a better housing solution for the unmarried respiratory cripple than apartment or housekeeping room arrangements, if the individual is willing to forgo his independence and adequate out-of-home care facilities are available. Such housing not only reduces the physical effort required in daily living but provides the presence of other persons in the event of an emergency. The problem of drinking which is manifested by some pulmonary cripples is not true alcoholism in all instances, but rather the undiscriminating man's way out of loneliness and fright and despair. Suitable congregate living arrangements, if desirable facilities exist, may decrease such emotional problems and thereby promote better health.

If this form of living arrangement is rejected by the recipient when it is first suggested, he may well have changed his mind at the time of the next visit, because his disability is progressive and by this time he may be more debilitated, or frightened about living alone. Consequently, the way should be left open for him to change his mind.

DIET

Because loss of weight and malnutrition are common problems, diet is an important item in preventing needless disability. Palatability of food is essential if the recipient is to be tempted to eat. More leeway for individual preferences may be permitted by a special diet allowance. If so, the worker may want to discuss the matter with the physician.

The single person may eat more if his budget permits restaurant meals than if he has to do his own cooking.

He may need to vary his eating plans to keep interested in food. When heart disease adds its own complications to the diet, an out-of-home care arrangement may provide the only solution for recipients who are single. The low-sodium diet, commonly known as "salt-free," is notorious for unpalatability, so that the recipient may well need the worker's help in finding means to secure adequate nutrition. The worker, in turn, may need to get help from the public health nutritionist or nurse, a clinic dietitian, or home economist with the agriculture department.

COUGHING

Tenacious sputum may create employment, housing, and social problems for some people. Coughing up a mass of phlegm after many throat-clearing efforts is unfortunately noisy, and the sound is unpleasant. Some clients, who have been made to feel repulsive to others or who are sensitive in this regard, find social contacts, group recreation, and church attendance embarrassing, and therefore withdraw. Those who have the physical strength to work at sedentary or light occupations may become too discouraged to do so.

The individual whose coughing occurs primarily when he first gets up in the morning has a different problem from the one who coughs unpredictably during the day. Consequently, the area is one which should be explored with the client if the worker has some clue that it confronts the client with a realistic problem.

SECURITY

It is difficult to give security to a recipient who has constantly recurring emergency needs and who tends to be fearful and upset. Social workers and physicians sometimes become impatient with clients who are always creating problems. An unfortunate tendency exists to belittle the problems of persons who cause us constant trouble, or to retaliate against the frightened, "difficult" person. But the punitive approach obviously makes matters worse.

A person who knows that his needs are accepted and understood, and who has learned which ones can be met and how, will feel more settled and secure than one who never knows where he stands, or who is made to feel that he has to prove how badly off he is to get anything. An understanding worker who is willing to put herself out to help the recipient with the details of his regimen and who provides a steadying influence makes an important contribution to the medical care of the individual. She is providing psychotherapy of the most valuable sort.

RECREATION AND RELIGIOUS INTERESTS

Relaxation and freedom from tension contribute to the patient's sense of well-being and are thus preventative or remedial measures. As with persons who have other crippling conditions, the pulmonary cripple profits from activity which keeps his mind off himself and brings a sense of pleasure. Television offers the best over-all solution, although many persons can also achieve relaxation from creative hobbies, reading, sedentary volunteer activities, card playing, shut-in club work, and so on.

Great peace of mind comes to those who are able to receive meaningful help from their religion. The anxious pulmonary cripple may benefit particularly from this help but find going to church difficult for various reasons connected with his disability and financial state. If the client seems to respond with interest when a question about church is raised, the worker should attempt to help him overcome practical problems in attending the church of his choice.

TERMS FREQUENTLY USED IN MEDICAL REPORTS

Barrel chest. A deformity resulting from chronic difficulty in expulsion of air from the lungs; an objective sign of advanced emphysema.

Bleb. Any bulla or vesicle filled with fluid.

Bronchodilator. A drug which dilates the bronchi.

Bronchogram. An X ray of the lungs after an opaque dye has been instilled into the bronchi.

Bronchoscopy. An examination of the bronchi through an instrument with a small light attached. The procedure is unpleasant for the patient and is usually dreaded. It is usually performed in the operating room of a hospital.

Bullae. Blisters in the lungs which are filled with air.

Cor pulmonale. Heart disease caused by disease of the lungs or of their blood vessels; an indication of far advanced lung disease and of poor prognosis.

Cyanosis. Blueness of the skin; an indication of insufficient oxygen in the blood.

Dyspnea. Difficult or labored breathing.

Epinephrine. A common bronchodilator drug.

Expiration-inspiration measurement. The measurement of the difference in chest size on breathing in and breathing out shows whether the chest is flexible or has become fixed in an expanded position. The usual healthy difference in measurement is five to six inches.

M.B.M. (maximum breathing capacity). A test which gives an index of ventilatory capacity of the lungs and presents an objective measurement of breathing reserve.

Orthopnea. Inability to breathe except in an upright position.

Pneumoconiosis. A chronic fibrous reaction in the lungs due to the inhalation of dust.

Polycythemia. An excess number of red blood cells, a disease condition which sometimes develops from chronic struggle for air.

Positive pressure; intermittent positive pressure. An oxygen treatment by machine for emphysema. The machine may be referred to as IPPB (intermittent positive pressure breathing) or as a Bennet Valve machine, after its designer.

Pulmonary. Pertaining to the lungs.

Pulmonary (or respiratory) cripple. A person who is too short of breath, because of lung damage, to function normally.

Rales. Abnormal sounds in the lungs heard through the stethoscope and indicating a pathologic condition. Rales are distinguished as dry or moist, according to the absence or pressure of fluid in the air passages, and are classified according to their location as bronchial, cavernous, laryngeal, pleural, tracheal, or vesicular.

Roentgenogram. An X ray.

Vital capacity. The amount of air the lungs can expel. A vital capacity test is frequently used as a measurement of the extent of crippling that has taken place because of damage to lung tissue.

CHAPTER VII

Progressive Diseases
of the Nervous System

THE NERVOUS SYSTEM is subject to a wide variety of disorders. Many are chronic, progressive, and severely disabling, denying their victims an opportunity for self-support and self-care and bringing them to the attention of the public assistance agency. Some of the disorders begin in early childhood, others in middle age, and some in later life.

The social and emotional toll taken by the degenerative neurological diseases is large. Although no treatment is available now to prevent their progression, symptoms can sometimes be temporarily controlled or slowed down and effects minimized by the joint efforts of doctor, social worker, and patient. The worker's activities have further importance in their significance for the client's family, because of what she can do to alleviate burden and suffering and to prevent family breakdown.

In addition to the chronic progressive neurological diseases, many of which are rare, other more common affections of the brain are relatively static. The aftereffects of cerebral vascular accidents (strokes) form the largest number. Epilepsy and cerebral palsy are also relatively static conditions.

Poliomyelitis is an example of an acute infection, sometimes followed by permanent crippling; encephalitis is another. The brain and spinal cord are also subject to accidents and tumors. The static, acute, or traumatic neurological disorders are discussed in separate chapters, because their social implications are different from each other and from those of the progressive conditions.

General Medical Base for Social Planning

PHYSIOLOGY

An outstanding account of the nervous system specifically written for social workers exists in Dr. Irving Berlin's articles on neurology published in *Social Casework* in November and December, 1956.* Since the details are readily accessible, they will not be repeated here.

Briefly, the nervous system is the governing agency of the body, controlling all muscular movements, internally responsible for all thoughts and for many of man's vital processes such as circulation and respiration. It receives stimuli through the sensory endings of the sense organs, conducts them to the brain where they are correlated and analyzed, and redistributes them as activities or reactions by means of the motor neurons which have their nerve endings in the muscles. Thus, man jumps when pricked by a pin, or speaks when spoken to.

---

* Irving Berlin, N.M.D., "A Review of Some Elements of Neurology," *Social Casework* XXXVII (Nov.–Dec., 1956), 427–433, 493–500.

The exquisitely refined, vital tissues of the central nervous system do not replace themselves once they have been destroyed. When damaged, the outlying nerves recover only very slowly. This explains why neurological disorders are so often incurable.

The nervous system includes the brain, spinal cord, twelve pairs of nerves arising from the brain stem (cranial nerves), thirty-one pairs from the spinal cord, and the nerves of the autonomic nervous system which supply the internal organs and blood vessels. The nerves are many neurons bound together, either sensory or motor; the cord is a tube made up of nerve cells and roots which relays impulses to the brain and back again to the muscles and also correlates simple reflexes; the brain is composed of the stem, the cerebellum, and the cerebrum, the latter being composed of two hemispheres and thought of as having five lobes.

The brain and cord are covered with three thin membranes (*meninges*). The space between the two closest to the brain tissue is filled with spinal fluid. There are three main cavities or *ventricles* in the brain (not to be confused with the ventricles of the heart), also filled with fluid, and communicating with each other and with the spaces between the meningeal covering of the brain and cord.

The function of the brain is so complex that it is not completely understood. Complicated acts, as for example picking up a pencil and writing with it, require a number of separate capacities, such as sight, recognition of objects, muscle action, coördination, thinking, memory, and use of language. The different parts of the brain must therefore work together.

In spite of the necessary relatedness of the brain's activities different parts have special functions. For example, the cerebellum, in the back part of the skull, correlates actions of muscle groups. A disturbance or disease affecting the cerebellum therefore produces lack of coördination and may cause staggering or tremors.

The hypothalamus, which was discussed in connection with the psychosomatic concept, and which lies in the mid-brain, is the center for integrating sensations with the basic emotions. However, the largest area of the brain—the cerebrum—is the area in which sensory experiences are blended and are associated with the higher functions of emotional control, reasoning, and judgment. Different lobes of the cerebrum have different functions; the occipital lobes in the back receive and sort out visual impressions, whereas the frontal lobes perform some of the most complex functions, such as reasoning, and also contain the speech center. Thus an injury to the occipital lobes could cause blindness, and one to a frontal lobe, loss of speech. The cranial nerves also have special functions—for example, II with sight, VIII with hearing.

Neurological testing relates to the form and structure of the brain as well as to the functions of its parts. It is obvious that a disease or injury which affects a certain part of the brain will be reflected in impaired function of specific parts or activities of the body. This well-known fact determines the method and terminology of a neurological examination. The skilled neurologist can locate a lesion in the brain by performing tests designed to reveal coördination and the capacity for skilled acts; by observing gait, abnormal movements, reflexes, muscle strength or weakness, nerve status, sensory responses; in some instances, by X-raying the skull or injecting air and X-raying the brain (*pneumoencephalogram*); by examining the spinal fluid by spinal tap; and by recording the electrical impulses of the brain (*electroencephalogram*—EEG).

Since the skull is rigid, increased pressure on the brain

results when a tumor is present, when an infection produces inflammation, when there is bleeding, or when an injury indents the skull. By the drawing off of spinal fluid, variations in pressure can be measured. By injection of an opaque substance into the spinal column and X ray of the cord (*myelogram*), any distortions in shape or sites of blockage can be found.

MULTIPLE SCLEROSIS

Some nerve cells are encased in a fatty covering (*myelin*). Patchy disintegration of this substance (*demyelination*), with replacement by scar tissue—*sclerosis*—scattered throughout the central nervous system, causes one of the most widely known of the degenerative diseases of the nervous system; multiple sclerosis or *"MS."*

Why the myelin breaks down is still unknown. The incidence of multiple sclerosis is highest in cold climates. The disease usually begins between the ages of twenty and forty. The individual often lives for fifteen to twenty-five years after onset.

The most unique feature of multiple sclerosis is that the symptoms can affect almost any part or function of the body, depending on where in the central nervous system the demyelinated patches occur. Another usual characteristic is the disappearance of the initial symptoms for an unpredictable period of time. Even after the disease is well established, the symptoms often become unpredictably better and then worse. The tendency to spontaneous remission (apparent arrest or cure) is one reason why persons with this disease are easy prey to quacks. If spontaneous remission coincides with a new treatment, however ineffectual or peculiar, the patient may think that the treatment caused the cure and enthusiastically endorse it to other MS victims of his acquaintance.

Symptoms most frequently include impaired vision, weakness of one or more limbs, lack of coördination, slurred speech, and bladder and bowel weakness. A frequent group of symptoms is shimmering movements of the eyeballs (*nystagmus*), *intention tremor* of the arms and hands, and slurred speech. Emotional instability, with either excessive cheerfulness (*euphoria*) or depression, is a common result of the disease.

The course, as indicated, may be marked by long plateaus with relatively little or only episodic impairment during the early years of the disease. In some cases, however, the condition is acute and steadily and rapidly worsens. Some persons live out a usual life span; others die in a few years with mental deterioration, blindness, and complete paralysis before death. Urinary incontinence or retention during advanced disease is among the most common distressing symptoms. Urinary infections can be serious and must be treated promptly. Fortunately, there are specific drugs which relieve these problems in many patients.

Treatment is now limited to general hygienic and supportive measures, drugs for relief of symptoms and infection, and sometimes physiotherapy to keep muscles in condition. A specialist whose interests lie in patient care can devise many small methods of ameliorating discomforts and handicaps.

Emotional upsets seem often to precipitate either the onset or progression of multiple sclerosis. Good morale seems to minimize the symptoms, so that all those things which give the patient a feeling of hope and comfort are physically as well as emotionally beneficial. Chilling, physical strain, and exhaustion are, like emotional upsets, likely to make the individual symptomatically worse.

The social worker should be actively involved in helping the client carry out the medical treatment plan, since good nutrition, financial provision for medical supervision and drugs, satisfactory housing and sleeping facilities, transportation to physiotherapy and occupational therapy centers, provision for recreation and stimulation, adequate warmth of clothing and housing, provision of appliances, and amelioration of personal or family problems constitute the bulk of the "general hygienic and supportive measures" which the doctor prescribes. A hopeful attitude and positive approach should be employed.

MUSCULAR DYSTROPHIES AND ATROPHIES

There are a number of muscular dystrophies and atrophies, most of them uncommon. They are caused by impairment or destruction of certain cells in the cord or brain. Why they develop is not known. They cannot be cured by any means known at this time. Much of what has been said about multiple sclerosis applies to these conditions.

It is impractical to try to remember the variations among the diagnoses. It is important, however, to recognize the names as indicating slowly progressive, wasting, incurable conditions; to know that their variations have great practical importance in social planning; and to find out from the physician and medical texts what the specific condition is likely to do to a given patient.

The most widely known is *muscular dystrophy* (MD), a hereditary condition usually beginning early in childhood or adolescence and usually terminating in death before adulthood. This slowly and steadily progressive disease is characterized by increasing muscle weakness and contractures.

AMYOTONIA CONGENITA

This childhood disease is characterized by progressive muscle weakness, and ends in death more quickly than does muscular dystrophy. The condition is rare, fortunately, and is probably congenital.

MYOTONIA ATROPHICA

A somewhat similar disease affecting adults is also hereditary and slowly progressive. It is characterized by wasting of muscles of the shoulder, face, legs, and feet. Patients with this disease have cataracts which sometimes have to be removed.

PROGRESSIVE MUSCULAR ATROPHY, SYRINGOMYELIA, AND AMYOTROPHIC LATERAL SCLEROSIS

These other painless, incurable neurological diseases cause progressive weakness and wasting of the extremities. Amyotrophic lateral sclerosis develops rapidly, and affects talking, swallowing, and the function of the arms and legs; death occurs within a few years. The course of progressive muscular atrophy and syringomyelia is long and slow.

The disease is familial. This fact adds to the emotional complications especially since there are sometimes several patients in one family. It and *Friedreich's Ataxia* usually begin earlier than the others.

MYASTHENIA GRAVIS

This is one of the more common of the slowly progressive neurological diseases and, like multiple sclerosis, is characterized by flare-ups and spontaneous periods of arrest or apparent cure. The muscle weakness (*myasthenia*) often occurs in the eyelids first, causing dropped lids (*ptosis*), which makes the person look sleepy, or it may be severe enough to create the same effects as blindness even though there is no defect of vision. The face muscles and throat muscles are also involved, causing life-threatening difficulty in swallowing and breathing.

The distinctive and important feature of this disease is that drugs (neostigmine, prostigmin, and related medications) exist which dramatically reverse the muscle weakness in many cases. The dropped eyelids quickly come back into place, the open mouth closes, strength returns to the weak limbs. The treatment is not a cure, but does permit an otherwise dangerously and severely disabled person to live an almost normal life. Consequently, it is urgent that social workers mark the words "myasthenia gravis" in their minds, and make sure that their clients with this disease have a way to get and keep taking the medicine which is restoring and lifesaving in so many cases.

In some instances surgery for removal of the thymus gland has been found effective, but this very serious operation should be performed only in major treatment centers.

HUNTINGTON'S CHOREA

This disease, another familial degenerative neurological condition which social workers usually encounter sooner or later, creates severe problems because pronounced mental impairment accompanies the physical symptoms. The person gradually develops, over a period of several years, involuntary irregular movements of the face, head, and hands, with progressive dementia.

Institutional care usually becomes necessary, because the burden of care is great. This disease, like most of the other familial neurological disorders, does not show up until early middle life.

PARKINSON'S DISEASE

Also known as "shaking palsy" or Paralysis agitans, this disease is familiar to social workers as a condition of later life in which the limbs shake while in relaxation (*resting tremor*) and the individual's face, body, and joints develop a progressive rigidity.

The cause of Parkinson's disease is obscure. It is not hereditary, nor is it due to hardening of the arteries. The fine tremor which some elderly persons develop simply as a result of arteriosclerosis should not be mistaken for Parkinson's disease. The disease is occasionally encountered in young persons as a result of encephalitis (the so-called sleeping sickness).

A socially significant fact is that emotional stress or physical exhaustion frequently triggers the first symptoms of Parkinson's disease, just as it does diabetes and rheumatoid arthritis, and, as in these diseases, anxiety and stress make the symptoms worse.

The symptoms themselves have special social significance: the shaking creates embarrassment, and the fatigue tends to create social isolation and depression. The difficulty of interviewing a constantly shaking person can make us appreciate how others must feel who have to be with him for a period of time, and how he must feel about the rejection he senses in others because of their discomfort.

The rigid facial muscles create a blank look similar to that of stupidity and a tendency to drool. Here again the symptoms invite rebuff, and consequently add to the suffering of the patient, thus by a vicious circle aggravating the already existing symptoms. The tiny steps and lack of balance that are a result of well-developed Parkinson's disease cause the individual to develop a curious running gait (*festination*) and inability to stop.

Parkinson's disease, like the other degenerative neurological disorders, cannot be cured, and is characterized by a long downhill course, frequently rapid for the first few years and then leveling off, so that the individual who has good medical and nursing care can live for many years, often dying eventually of some other immediate cause. However, the need for help with the ordinary activities of daily living is obvious. Diet and nutrition need careful medical supervision, because severe complications can grow out of constipation caused by the disease.

Various measures can be undertaken materially to reduce the severity of the symptoms. Certain drugs are helpful, artane and hyoscine being among those commonly used. Physiotherapy is likewise of considerable ameliorative value. Skilled neurosurgery on the brain can halt the symptoms temporarily in certain selected patients. Although it is estimated that not more than 15 per cent are good candidates for neurosurgery, the possibility of surgical help in this disease should not be forgotten.

The simple psychotherapy which can be provided by doctor, social worker, and family is an important factor in overcoming the depression and anxiety which make symptoms worse. Reduction of insecurity, emotional support, cheerful surroundings, opportunities for escape into recreation or interests, cultivation of religious resources, and a hopeful outlook are vital adjuncts to the medical aids prescribed by the doctor. Adaptation of clothing and furniture to reduce frustration and dependency also relieves depression and is therefore a part of the medical-social treatment.

Implications for Public Assistance

The neurological degenerative diseases have many similarities, but the differences are important in social planning.

Thus, the social worker needs to read about the specific diagnosis which has been made in order to secure a general background, and then to find out from the doctor the answers to a number of questions.

MEDICAL QUESTIONS

Is this generally a slowly developing or a rapidly developing disease? Is it characterized by steady downhill progression, or do long plateaus exist? In other words, what can the client and social worker expect in regard to continuing capacity for employment, household occupation, and the pursuit of former interests? Is the disease one in which the upper or the lower extremities are normally involved first, or are either or both ever involved? Are the muscles involved those which determine fine movements or gross movements? Is coördination normally impaired? What about vision, speech, swallowing?

We want also to know whether exercise or activity of the muscles is harmful, as it definitely is in some diseases. Is it necessary to guard against deformities? If so, how should this be done—for example, by physiotherapy, footboards on the bed, boards under the mattress, proper use of pillows, proper height of chairs, attention to posture?

Are there any medicines which help alleviate symptoms —as in myasthenia gravis, Parkinson's disease, or the relief of incontinence in multiple sclerosis? Are the symptoms dangerous—as, for example, weakness of breathing or swallowing muscles? Are there certain things to be avoided—such as exercise, infections, chilling, overfatigue?

Is the client near the end of his life, or does the doctor estimate that he still has a number of years ahead? How much has the doctor told the patient? Has the doctor discussed the prognosis with a family member? If not, will he do so if an appointment can be arranged?

Once the medical picture has been obtained, the worker and client can plan accordingly. It must be remembered that the physician may often decide not to reveal to the client the hopeless nature of the disease, and therefore the worker may work under the handicap of knowing considerably more than she may reveal to the client.

The questions as to which categorical aid is appropriate —whether a vocational rehabilitation referral is worth while, what special needs should be planned for in the budget, whether housing needs to be improved, whether devices such as ramps and bathroom rails need to be considered, whether nursing home placement will enter the picture, how appropriate the client's depression or elation may be—are all dependent upon the answers to the questions which have been raised with the physician.

COMMON PROBLEMS

Public assistance planning frequently needs to take into account: a long, slow downhill course with its anxiety and discouragement; a tendency of the rehabilitation agency to find the client "not feasible" medically; a problem of urinary incontinence in late stages, with its spirit-breaking implications; the increasing burden on the family of increasing invalidism of a formerly active member; the need for maximum nutrition and bodily resistance; the need, as the disease progresses, for appliances and devices and for a comfortable and medically appropriate bed and chair.

The long, slow downhill course is a source of overpowering anxiety to both patient and family, especially in those instances where other family members have had the same disease or where the patient knows other persons with the same diagnosis whose condition is more advanced than his. The dread of, and then the horror of, finding oneself unable to walk, eat, get out of bed, take care of one's toilet needs, has been graphically described by articulate patients. The normal reaction is depression. In some instances the anxiety is so great that it cannot be faced, and by a peculiar psychological reaction the patient assumes an unnatural cheerfulness (*euphoria*). When this occurs the client can be misleading, insisting that everything is fine when in truth great need exists. No effort should be made to force the patient to face the truth about his condition; needless to say, however, necessary protective measures may have to be taken for some other, ostensible reason.

False reassurance is unwise in working with clients suffering from an overwhelming, realistic anxiety. If the individual can talk to a quiet perceptive listener who understands how he feels, who briefly commends him for his courage, accepts the naturalness of his feelings, and does what he can to relieve the practical difficulties, this is more helpful than "pep" talks or the injection of false hopes.

Spiritual resources are often meaningful to persons with progressively crippling conditions. Church attendance can often be arranged, even for wheel-chair patients, through the clergyman or church members. A proper suit or dress to wear to church, and the ability to put a coin on the collection plate, obviously are important to the client in these instances.

The ability to get outdoors and to go places, such as to the grocery store, library, clinic, and movies, or to go for automobile rides, is of great importance in helping the person forget himself, find new things to think about, shorten the days, and feel himself a normal part of the human race. Living on the first floor assumes major importance for an individual with impaired strength in the lower extremities, as do ramps when a wheel-chair existence becomes necessary.

Television needs hardly to be mentioned as the greatest

possible help to anxiety-ridden and invalided persons. When sets need repair or have been taken back by the company for lack of payments, it is usually possible to have repairs made or to obtain a new set through a small charitable group of some kind, since the kindness of the gift is so obvious.

The tendency of the rehabilitation agency to find the client "not feasible" for vocational rehabilitation is to be expected in light of the prognosis in many instances. The client should be spared the unnecessary discouragement and feeling of rejection which an adverse decision brings, if the decision can be anticipated. Therefore, it is well to talk with the doctor first, find out the medical possibilities, and then discuss the situation with the vocational rehabilitation service before mentioning it to the client.

If the rehabilitation service does not accept the client, home employment or selling, occupational therapy, and adult education classes afford the early neurological cripple important avenues for losing himself in useful and creative activity. Budgeting should provide for transportation, and necessary clothing, fees, and financial incentive for effort when policy permits.

The several problems of physical deterioration, such as incontinence, increasing burden on the family, need for maximum nutrition and for appliances and devices, all indicate the need for the help which a public health nurse or visiting nurse can provide. Needless to say, she is better able than the social worker to plan with the doctor and the client the kind of equipment the client needs, and to teach him how to take care of it and himself. Mechanical aids can greatly reduce small physical problems with large emotional implications, but they need to be worked out carefully and in an individualized fashion by someone who has had experience with them. Further, money spent for good quality equipment may be wasted if the client has not been taught how to use the devices and therefore does not use them.

The social worker will need to remain active in the case even though the nurse too is calling. The client's feelings about his physical condition—feelings of resentment, fear, humiliation, despair, or anxiety—may be so great that he responds poorly to the nurse's efforts. She may even consider him dull, stubborn, or uncoöperative, and perhaps abandon her efforts in favor of someone who uses her services more effectively. Thus, the worker needs to keep in touch with the nurse and, if possible, to arrange a conference. Pooling information and ideas and giving expression to discouragement to each other often make a fresh start possible.

When incontinence adds to the personal and family burden imposed by neurological disease, matters of laundry and sufficient supplies should be explored. As a mother's feelings about the burden of an infant is lessened by a sufficient number of diapers to avoid undue fatigue and inconvenience, so is a homemaker's feelings about an invalid influenced by the ease or difficulty of laundry. The supply of sheets and the repair of the washing machine are important. The client's ability to keep clean is obviously paramount for his feeling of self-respect, his ability to be accepted by others, and, when he is ambulatory, for his opportunities for occupation.

Except where the physician has become concerned by the patient's malnutrition, he may not think about the need to request a special diet. (Some doctors think of an ordinary diet as what they themselves have at home.) The physician may welcome a clue from the social worker that tempting, palatable, easily digested food will be more readily available to the recipient if he recommends a high-vitamin, high-protein diet. Food is important in maintaining morale as well as the best possible physical condition.

By attention to the recipient's morale and nutritional state, he can be kept up and around as long as possible, thus reducing the burden on the family. When he does become invalided, some regular relief for the caretaker should be explored. Help from volunteers or relatives sometimes can be obtained. If not, policy may permit allowance in the assistance grant for this service.

TERMS FREQUENTLY USED IN MEDICAL REPORTS

Achilles reflex. Ankle jerk test.

Aphonia. Loss of voice.

Ataxia. Failure of muscular coördination.

Atrophy. Wasting away, with diminution in size.

Babinski sign. A neurological test. The big toe jerks up and the other toes curl in when the underside of the foot is stroked.

Cerebellar. Pertaining to the cerebellum, the lower part of the brain, which controls movements.

Cerebral. Pertaining to the cerebrum, the main or top part of the brain, divided into two "hemispheres" and controlling the higher functions, such as reasoning.

Cranial. Pertaining to the head or cranium.

Diplopia. Double vision.

Dura mater. The outermost of the three meninges or coverings of the brain.

Dysarthria. Imperfect articulation in speech.

Dystrophy. Degeneration or wasting.

Electroencephalogram (EEG). Painless test of electrical activity in the brain.

Euphoria. Unwarranted, excessive cheerfulness.

Festination. A running gait.

Fossa. A hollow place or depression. The cerebral fossae are the declivities in the cranium which hold the brain lobes.

Glia. Neurological substance in one of the layers in the brain.

Hyperreflexia. Overactive reflexes.

Intention tremor. Tremor occurring when the individual begins a movement of the muscles involved.

Meninges. Membranes covering the brain.

Myasthenia. Muscle weakness.

Myelin. Fatty sheath around some nerves.

Nystagmus. Shimmering movement of the eyeballs.

Parasthesia. A peculiar sensation.

Pneumoencephalogram. Test involving injection of air into the skull.

Ptosis. Dropped eyelids (pronounced *tōsĭs*); can also refer to dropping of an organ or part.

Resting tremor. Tremor occurring when muscle is at rest.

Romberg test. A test of coördination in which the subject stands with his eyes closed and feet together. The amount of swaying is noted.

Ventricle. Hollow chamber.

CHAPTER VIII

Epilepsy

EPILEPSY is a condition characterized by recurrent paroxysms in which an impairment of consciousness occurs, and which may or may not be accompanied by convulsive movements of the body. There are three common forms: *grand mal,* in which the individual has major convulsions; *petit mal,* in which he is subject to lapses of consciousness with either slight or no convulsive movements; *psychomotor* epilepsy, in which there are seizures not of convulsions but of psychic phenomena and abnormal behavior.

Some epileptics have seizures which come only at night—nocturnal, rather than diurnal, attacks. For this reason, and also because many have their seizures well under control and do not mention them, the number of epileptics in the population is much larger than often realized, being estimated at about one person in every two hundred of the population.

Seizures usually begin during infancy or adolescence. In

acquired cases, they may begin any time after a head injury—even many years later. Some children outgrow seizures. Therefore, the aid-to-dependent-children workers and child-welfare workers are probably most likely to be concerned with epilepsy, although the adult epileptic may be found in every caseload.

It is estimated that in 75 per cent of the cases most of the convulsions can be brought under control by proper dosages of medication. Frequently the informed physician can work a miracle in the client's life by bringing about almost complete control. The social worker has the joy of seeing relative normalcy replace severe disability as a reward for her efforts in getting the client under adequate medical care.

The tragedy in the situation is that many persons, for lack of knowledge or resources, do not receive needed medical care. Some of these become mentally impaired from too many severe convulsions before adequate treatment is instituted. Even if physical normalcy is achieved, many cannot achieve social normalcy because of the attitude of the community and because of personality damage that has already occurred. However, the social challenge of working with epileptics is very great, because in no disease does one find more social problems, many of which are amenable to at least some amelioration.

General Medical Base for Social Planning

In former years a sharp distinction was drawn between acquired epilepsy, caused by an injury to the brain, and epilepsy the person was born with, *idiopathic* epilepsy (of unknown origin). At present it is believed that all epilepsy is the result of a congenitally low threshold toward convulsions and some form of injury, the proportion of the mixture of the two varying from a relatively low threshold with a slight injury to a high threshold and a severe injury. However, the existence of an old injury cannot be pinpointed in most cases, which are therefore still called idiopathic.

Epilepsy is familial in terms of low thresholds for convulsions, but there is less danger of inheritance than formerly thought. It is inherited only when there exists a family history of epilepsy or migraine on both maternal and paternal sides. Various items influence the likelihood of inheritance, such as the age the convulsions began in the parent (the later the better from this standpoint). Although there is no "average" case, the figures quoted by the National Epilepsy League indicate that the epileptic parent has one chance in forty of having an epileptic child.* However, such wide variations exist in regard to the inheritance factor that a consultation with a physician is desirable when an epileptic is considering marriage and progeny.

PHYSIOLOGY

Epileptic seizures occur because of the manner in which electrical impulses of the brain are discharged. Certain clusters of nerve cells may give off an autonomous discharge, instead of waiting until they receive an appropriate stimulus, and cause a paroxysmal, abnormal activity in the brain. The rebel clusters responsible which have been identified thus far are at the edges of a "scar" from some sort of injury, infection, or hemorrhage. It is presumed that those which cannot be identified are similar but in inaccessible parts of the brain.

When a person has a predisposition to seizures, or a con-

* William G. Lennox, M.D., "Marriage and Children for Epileptics," *Human Fertility* X (Dec., 1945).

genitally low threshold for convulsions, his brain wave pattern is usually, though not always, distinctive and consequently can be identified by an *electroencephalogram* (EEG), a painless test in which brain wave patterns are recorded on a piece of graph paper. Seizures do not always mean epilepsy—they can be due to a variety of causes. It is important for those who have seizures to have a diagnostic examination at the best available facility.

Persons who do have paroxysmal abnormal activity in the brain respond to excitement or ill health or lowered resistance by having a seizure; a person with a normal brain wave pattern might react to the same stimulus by a different response, such as turning white, showing anger, crying, or manifesting a variety of reactions depending on the personality.

An *aura* (warning of impending seizures), occurring in many patients, is an important feature from a social standpoint, because it gives the person a chance to get out of harm's way, making more flexibility possible in his occupation and recreation and lessening the need for constant supervision. The aura is said to consist of various kinds of subjective phenomena, such as feeling nauseated, smelling a strange odor, seeing lights.

TREATMENT

The treatment of epilepsy consists primarily of administering anticonvulsant drugs and of reducing the precipitating factors of emotional stress and low bodily resistance. Occasionally brain surgery is indicated to remove a scar, but this drastic measure is not undertaken if treatment by drugs is successful. It can be done only if scars have been identified in an accessible part of the brain.

The anticonvulsant drugs are fortunately very effective, once the right dosage and the right combination have been worked out for the individual patient. The most common of these drugs at the present time are phenobarbital, dilantin, mesantoin, and tridione. Finding the right combination requires skill and experience on the part of the doctor, as well as patience over a period of trial and error. The client too must have patience, and a means of transportation, and an understanding of what is going on, if he is to keep on returning to the clinician while the latter is working out the dosage.

Once the medication has been determined, the patient has to stay under supervision. Some of the drugs have toxic side effects, and a modification of dosage may be needed. For example, dilantin given in large doses over a long period can cause hypertrophy (an unhealthy proliferation of tissues) of the gums which may require oral surgery.

The patient also needs to be active. Mental and physical exercise and well-being are important in achieving control of seizures. These requirements may be difficult to achieve because of the personal problems epilepsy causes.

Grand mal seizures are, of course, highly dangerous, particularly those which occur without an aura. Loss of sphincter control, urinary and bowel, occurs. Some persons with epilepsy are intensely fearful of falling. Many find social contacts painful because of the possible embarrassment of having a seizure in front of others. These feelings and fears are rational and realistic.

Social workers are not called upon to give physical care to a client in a seizure; but if a client has a seizure in the worker's presence, she should help to dispel curious onlookers and to get him to a quiet place where he can rest for as long as necessary after the seizure, since he may be drowsy and unfit to take care of himself for several hours. A person in a psychomotor seizure of aberrant behavior should not be unnecessarily restrained, because this increases violence; rather, he should be protected for a short period, and then helped to get home safely.

The problems which interfere with effective treatment are, broadly speaking, social in nature. Not every community has a doctor interested in the treatment of epilepsy, and the patient may need to go to a specialist. The anticonvulsant drugs have to be taken conscientiously every day, and the uninteresting, undramatic matter of constant pill taking seems to be difficult for most persons. Medical supervision and drugs may cost more than the family can pay, or, in a month when other expenses are high, the family may feel that medical care is the only item which can be put off.

In cases that are difficult to control, so much medicine may have to be taken, at least for an experimental period, that the patient may become drowsy and stupid. He may be so lethargic that he requires supervision to prevent accidents and also to see that he takes the pills on a regular schedule.

OUTLOOK

In a few cases, seizures in childhood lessen with age or the child "grows out of them." However, if grand mal seizures cannot be brought under control, the constantly recurring severe paroxysms may damage the brain. In some cases, the individual deteriorates, both physically and mentally, and ends in an institution or goes into *status epilepticus,* which is a state of constant seizures ending in death if the person cannot be brought out of them. Mental deterioration is fortunately not so common as generally supposed, seriously affecting only about 10 per cent of epileptics. The prognosis is usually better for those of normal mentality and mentally normal parents and for those who have not had a severe brain injury.

Epilepsy is rarely cured. The goal is life-long control of convulsions.

Implications for Public Assistance

Epileptics were once considered to be possessed of devils, and the cultural stigma still seems to hold. The disease creates many social and psychological problems. Epilepsy has been so long mistakenly associated with insanity, feeble-mindedness, alcoholism, and degeneration, that even social workers sometimes withdraw from working with an epileptic on the basis that he cannot be helped and is a fearsome person to be around.

MEDICAL AND SOCIAL EVALUATION

Epilepsy may mean only a small disability in an otherwise brilliant and productive person, or it may mean total deterioration. Such a wide variety of conditions exists that the first task of the social worker is to individualize the particular client and what the disease means in the particular case.

An early step is to get a history from someone other than the client, if there is someone available who knows him well. The epileptic often does not know how many seizures he has, what kind they are, how long he is incapacitated afterward, or when they began, because of the impairment of consciousness which occurs. Further, wittingly or unwittingly, he often minimizes the frequency and kind of seizures he has, because of the humiliation he feels about them.

The worker should know how often he has spells, and when they occur (day or night, regularly at certain times of day or the month, or sporadically), what kind they are, and whether he has a warning, in order to have any idea of what the client is up against and what, if any, aid he qualifies for.

Has the individual had the advantage of modern medical treatment, and is he regularly taking some of the new drugs? If not, there can be no assessment of what kind of situation or permanent disability will obtain until after the person has been placed under the best medical treatment available and is helped to obtain and regularly take the prescribed medicine. Several months may elapse before the physician will be able to make an estimate of how the person is going to respond to treatment. Most will respond well. If they are helped to take their drugs regularly and stay under care, they probably will not qualify for aid on the basis of physical disability alone.

However, they may find it impossible to get and hold a job. Most employers will not hire epileptics, or they discharge them after the first seizure on the job. Then too, the personality of the epileptic may have been so damaged by the disease itself, and/or by the stigma he felt, and the possible abnormal family relationships and unhappy school background he had, if any, that he is not fitted for employment. If he has been rejected and taunted from childhood and deprived of an education, as many epileptic children are, he may be too withdrawn and shy to relate to others, or so angry and emotional that his instability creates constant crises. Consequently, a comprehensive and thoughtful social history needs to be prepared for consideration of categorical aid or referral to vocational rehabilitation services. The "whole person" and his total disability should be taken into account.

EMPLOYMENT

Employment must be in a safe situation, and the job one not requiring the person to drive a car. This is of course true for any epileptic, even one under seemingly good control.

Unless such a job is available in the community, the "employable" epileptic will be unemployable. Helping the person to secure some type of useful activity, even if the remuneration is small, provides the best kind of psychotherapy. However, it may require extensive and repeated efforts. Sheltered workshop employment may be desirable if regular employment cannot be secured.

MENTAL IMPAIRMENT

The extent of mental impairment is often difficult to assess. Only a small percentage of epileptics are said to be retarded, but the effect of drugs may give that impression in many who are not. If there is a problem, the physician should be consulted about whether the final dosage has been determined or whether the person is still in the experimental dosage period, and whether there is hope that his condition can be controlled so as to have less drowsiness as a side effect. The physician may be prescribing the least expensive medication because of the client's finances; he may be able to substitute something less soporific if more expensive drugs can be allowed.

SOCIAL AND PSYCHOLOGICAL PROBLEMS

An unfortunate hazard for the low-income epileptic is being jailed for what is mistaken for drunkenness when he is in a stupor after a seizure. His phenobarbital may be removed from his possession by the police because it is a narcotic. Without his medicine, the individual may then be subject to seizures and even to status epilepticus. Some physicians advise as a precaution that all epileptics carry cards which give their diagnosis, physician's name, and their prescribed medicine.

Epileptics may also be robbed while they are unconscious. Money management measures such as provision of board and lodging may have to be undertaken for the protection of the individual with uncontrolled grand mal attacks.

The epileptic who is unable to find a job, subject to various indignities and lack of satisfying social relationships, may develop undesirable forms of escape, such as alcoholism, which further compound his social problems and worsens his physical condition.

The family relationships of the epileptic are often impaired. Parents may be rejecting or overprotective, or may have had an exhausting experience trying to help an epileptic child through the vicissitudes of growing up. They frequently feel defensive, thinking that the child's condition is a reflection on one of them. If the child or adult seeks to adjust by withdrawal and social isolation, the family may encourage this.

SOCIAL TREATMENT

What can the social worker do to help clients with such socially difficult disabilities? The first steps should be concentration on helping the individual receive the best possible medical treatment, and then upon a social situation which ensures that he takes his medicine regularly. Physician's visits, medication, and transportation for regular continuing medical care are frequently associated financial needs.

The social situation should be assessed with reference to general hygienic measures, in order to make sure that, if possible, the epileptic has the advantage of a good diet, regular hours, and a comfortable place to sleep. A board-and-care living arrangement may prove the most satisfactory if he has no family or if the family relationships are disturbing and cannot be rectified. A client who has serious personality difficulties may need to be placed in a specially licensed facility.

The factors that are especially disturbing to the epileptic

person should be understood, and any possible measures taken to alleviate them. These steps will reduce the number of seizures and, to the extent that they are successful, will clear away the worst obstacles to his maximum adjustment. Some forms of regular occupation, exercise, and social opportunities are so vitally important that they justify the time which is often required to work them out.

The casework relationships and counseling measures are also important and not easy. The worker must be prepared to use aggressive tactics to protect the client's interests if his condition is such that he needs to be shielded from harm or exploitation. She must also prepare to be a calm, stable anchor for the client and his family if he has personality problems and uncontrolled seizures resulting in frequent social crises.

The protective helping role may induce emotional dependency in the client if he has no other means of securing the comfort and pleasure of having someone on whom he can always rely. This dependency tends to be irksome, and tempts the worker to become irritable with the client for leaning too much. It can be minimized by limiting the length or frequency of interviews and at the same time by helping the client to secure other sources of security and appreciation through work, occupational therapy, church activities, the interest of clinical personnel, or improved family relationships.

TERMS FREQUENTLY USED IN MEDICAL REPORTS

Aura. A warning of an impending seizure through a sensation or bodily experience.

Dilantin. A recently discovered and excellent drug for the control of grand mal and psychomotor epilepsy. It may cause undesirable side effects, particularly damage to the gums, if taken in excessive amounts and consequently must be supervised closely.

Diurnal. Daily; referring to seizures that occur in the daytime.

EEG, electroencephalogram. A painless test wherein the electrical impulses of the brain are recorded and interpreted.

Epileptic equivalent. A seizure type corresponding to psychomotor epilepsy.

Grand mal. Literally large sickness; major convulsions.

Idiopathic. Of unknown origin.

Mesantoin. A new and effective medicine for epileptic seizures.

Nocturnal. Nightly; referring to seizures that occur at night.

Petit mal. Literally small illness; fleeting impairments of consciousness, often so slight as to be misinterpreted as mere lapses of attention.

Phenobarbital. One of the most common drugs for seizures, and one of the cheapest, but one which may make the individual drowsy and stupid if taken in large amounts.

Psychomotor. Describes seizures that combine psychic and bodily effects, ranging from small movements to violent behavior or antisocial acts.

Status epilepticus. A dangerous condition in which the person goes from one seizure into another without stopping. A medical emergency.

Tridione. A highly specific and effective drug to control petit mal seizures.

CHAPTER IX

Cerebral Palsy

CEREBRAL PALSY is a permanent neuromuscular disability, usually caused by prenatal or birth injury to the motor control centers of the brain. It may not only produce a lack of muscular control but frequently creates mental retardation, seizures, and other sensory and behavior disorders as well. The condition was formerly called Little's disease or spastic paralysis. The experts refer to it sometimes in specific descriptive terms such as *congenital diplegia,* or *spastic quadriplegia,* or *athetosis.*

The extent of the problem is not known, but it has been estimated that about one in every 200 children is brain injured and that there are about 400,000 adult cerebral palsied in the United States. The death rate among cerebral palsied is much higher than normal, although the condition is not progressive and should not cause death by itself. No social, geographic, or economic influences are known to affect the incidence of the condition. Since only a small percentage of the significantly handicapped cerebral palsied become employable, a proportionately large number may be expected on the rolls of the OASDI (childhood disability benefit) program and the public assistance agencies.

Many qualify for the aid to the disabled program in early adult life. Because most severely handicapped cerebral palsied do not marry, the adults will not constitute a large group in the aid to dependent children program. It seems to be uncommon to find people with cerebral palsy receiving old age assistance, but they may be receiving general assistance and living with parents who receive old age assistance.

The family and child welfare workers have an unusual opportunity to be of service to the cerebral palsied children in their caseloads, for treatment should begin in infancy or as early as possible.

The relative youth of the adults that come to the public assistance agency and the fact that their disability will not get worse impel us to concentrate upon alleviation of dependency and upon rehabilitation toward a more satisfying life even though complete self-support may be an unrealistic goal. The problems encountered are very great, requiring application of sufficient knowledge to make possible efforts that are selective and relevant.

General Medical Base for Social Planning

CAUSE

Cerebral palsy is not inherited. The brain damage which causes it is primarily the result of lack of oxygen to the brain of the fetus, with consequent tissue damage, during the prenatal period or during the birth process. The brain injury can occur in a variety of ways, such as illness of the mother during pregnancy, premature birth, breech birth, improper use of instruments by the obstetrician, precipitate birth, and so forth.

Because cerebral palsy is not curable and is indeed a grave burden for the individual and his family, all possible preventive efforts should be made. Social workers should concentrate particularly on helping pregnant women get the best possible prenatal and confinement care. More than a referral to a clinic is often necessary; getting there, baby-sitting arrangements for the other small children, transportation to the hospital when labor begins, and provision for special diet are some of the many problems with which the mother may need help.

The kind of cerebral palsy depends upon what part of the brain was injured; the severity of the crippling upon the severity of the damage. Damage to the brain stem permits unplanned movements to occur, either shudders or tremors or the twisting, purposeless, wormlike movements called *athetosis*. The athetoid cripple is frequently affected in arms, neck, and head; when he starts to make a movement with the upper part of his body, it may overflow to his trunk and legs.

This group of cerebral palsied is not so large as the so-called *spastic* group. Spastic paralysis, affecting about 60 per cent of the total, is caused by damage to the motor cortex of the brain. Stiffness and rigidity are the attributes of spasticity. These may occur on one side only—*spastic hemiplegia;* in the lower extremities only—*spastic paraplegia;* or all four extremities may be involved—*spastic quadriplegia.*

The individual with spastic paralysis usually holds his arm pressed against the body, the forearm bent at right angles to the upper arm, the fist clenched tightly. He may walk on his toes or outer part of the ball of the foot, with the leg turned inward and the knee bent. If both legs are involved, the tight muscles draw the legs together, pulling them inward at the hips, resulting in a *scissors* gait.

An important gain in understanding the physiology of spasticity (and therefore what is and what is not sensible in treatment) is the theory elucidated by the English neurologist Dr. Karel Bobath. He points out that in fulfilling its function of integration of motor behavior, the central nervous system affects muscles in groups and not single muscles. For example, at first a normal baby cannot make selective, fine movements but moves all over in reaching for something; as the baby matures, he learns to suppress or inhibit gross movements and to make only the fine movement intended.

Dr. Bobath and others believe that the lesions of cerebral palsy interfere with the inhibitory mechanisms; that because of the inability to suppress, the patient is left with gross movement patterns affecting the whole body. At the same time a derailment of automatic movement patterns occurs, leaving abnormal pattern reactions.

The emphasis on the fact that the dysfunction in movement and in speech is not due to local muscular weakness, but to abnormal coördination or abnormal patterns affecting the whole body, points to the uselessness and waste of funds in treating individual muscles. It also points to the fact that treatment or teaching the cerebral-palsied person a different pattern of movement should begin in infancy.

Various authorities, including Dr. Bobath, further emphasize that the whole child, not just his body, is affected and that he must therefore be treated as a whole. His perception of himself and the world may be different because of his crippling. Certainly the helplessness of the moderately or severely advanced cerebral-palsied keeps him dependent longer on his parents, more fearful, and less exposed to the learning experience of normal children.

The same lack of oxygen or other injury to the brain tissue that causes the muscle movement abnormalities often causes other problems. It is estimated that speech is affected (this may be because of muscular impairment or because of a brain communication defect) in 75 per cent of the cases, hearing in 15 per cent, vision in 50 per cent; and that a large number, perhaps 40 per cent, have convulsions.

Mental retardation is common, the estimates ranging to as much as 75 per cent. However, any figures on mental retardation must be examined with caution; intelligence tests do not test anything except what the individual has learned during his lifetime, and the severely handicapped child is often not exposed to normal learning situations, thus responding to tests with a low IQ.

The multiplicity of problems involved is one of the reasons why cerebral palsy creates such a severe disability.

TREATMENT

Treatment is predicated first on a careful individualization of the patient. Physical conditions vary from spasticity so mild that it can hardly be detected to complete invalidism. These conditions are accompanied by every gradation of mental capacity, concomitant physical problems, and by all degrees of emotional stability and motivation.

A comprehensive approach is essential when a condition is under consideration which is actually a complex rather than a single entity. The necessary individualization usually requires a variety of tests, including a social history, psychological tests, physical examination, hearing tests, vision tests, and muscle tests.

Mental testing ordinarily precedes treatment decisions, because the patient needs a certain mentality to coöperate. If the individual drools, twists his head, and speaks with a guttural voice, because of muscular problems, he often gives the impression of severe retardation which may not exist at all. The tests which rely on performing certain activities within a time limit cannot be used with many of the cerebral palsied, and those which are predicated on normal learning experiences cannot be accurately applied to an individual who has been kept indoors, given little stimulation, and not sent to school. Problems of vision and hearing may create additional barriers to adequate test results. Consequently the psychologist may need to secure advice or to refer the patient to someone with better facilities and wider experience in testing disabled persons. Frequently prolonged observation has to be substituted for testing.

After a relatively accurate psychological test has been made, the selection of the patient for medical treatment should be determined by stability and motivation as well as by intelligence. Experience has shown that a dull but better-motivated, more stable person will frequently respond better to treatment than a brighter but less stable person.

Because cerebral palsy cannot be cured, the objectives of treatment are to prepare the patient for maximum self-care, appearance of normalcy, and vocational opportunity. This frequently means special attention to speech therapy and to the use of the hands and arms, so that the individual can take care of himself and have adequate means of communicating with others. To be able to speak so that one can be understood is perhaps more important than any other activity. Approximating a normal appearance is an important goal, in order to develop normal relationships and thereby to secure maximum learning and working opportunities and emotional stability.

For many years professional debate has taken place as to the best methods of treating the cerebral-palsied, with different emphases upon exercises, bracing, and surgery.

The consensus seems to be that the individual can be truly helped only by years of relaxing and conditioning exercises begun as early as possible—ideally, in early infancy. (The expense is obviously very great.) However, bracing and surgery are sometimes necessary to prevent or correct certain deformities or to achieve stabilization.

Bracing may be used to support weak legs or trunks, to stretch out contractures, or to control wild motions as an aid in reducing conspicuousness.

Surgery to correct contractures or to prevent "scissoring" is wasteful if the balance of the affected muscles or tendons is such that the pulls will continue and cause the difficulty all over again. If the contracture is the result of some habitual posture rather than a pull, surgery is helpful. Therefore surgery should be decided upon carefully by a specialist.

Bone stabilizing operations on the feet and legs are sometimes used successfully, as are bone operations to correct twisting. Brain surgery to stop involuntary motion is in the process of development.

Braces, crutches, and wheel chairs are important in the treatment of the cerebral palsied as aids to ambulation and therefore to wider opportunities for self-care and independence. Any permanent or long-time cripple should have devices which are tailor-made to fit well and to produce as much support and comfort as possible.

Drugs are not a usual part of the appropriate treatment of the cerebral palsied unless he has epilepsy. In such cases, seizures are controlled in the same manner as are those of any epileptic. Tranquilizers are being used to aid relaxation in some cases. There is great progress in drug manufacture. Perhaps in the future we will find drugs of great benefit.

Implications for Public Assistance

Cerebral palsy varies so widely in extent and severity that its social ramifications are also wide. As in other conditions, individualization of the condition and what it means to the person is requisite to an intelligent social treatment plan. Mild cerebral palsy will usually create no great problems.

Moderate or severe cerebral palsy, with other accompanying handicaps, will, however, involve the social worker in certain recurring areas: medical care, special needs related to the various forms of therapy and to mechanical aids in daily living, education, employment, recreation, and family and psychological problems. The extremely handicapped recipient has additional special problems which should be taken into account when one is working with him and his family.

MEDICAL CARE

Achievement of maximum functioning—more properly called habilitation than rehabilitation—first requires the best physical condition which can be achieved. If the recipient did not have exercises for relaxation and control in infancy and childhood, he may still benefit to some extent from treatment during adult life; at any rate he should have the opportunity for professional evaluation of feasible treatment objectives. Objectives may be limited to improving only one small part of self-care or mobility, but even a limited improvement is worth while. The social worker should not pass judgment as to whether the recipient can benefit from treatment, needless to say, for his appearance and present level of attainment may be no gauge.

In many instances, inquiry will reveal that the recipient has had an evaluation, treatment, and special education through the crippled children's program and the school system. In such cases a summary should be secured in order to ascertain what the recipient's tests (psychological as well as physical) showed, what was done, and what the doctor recommended at the time treatment was discontinued. Past experience is often a valuable guide as to what may and may not be feasible now.

Because treatment of the cerebral palsied is so complex, it is fortunate that several resources exist for comprehensive evaluation. Available in most communities are: orthopedists and pediatricians in the crippled children's program (for recipients less than 21 years of age) and specialists connected with private crippled children's organizations and cerebral palsy associations, workshops and rehabilitation centers, and the vocational rehabilitation services.

Consequently, requests for authorization of treatments or braces usually need not be considered in a piecemeal manner. Nor should it be necessary to embark on physical restoration and social measures directed toward schooling, employment, institutional placement, attendant care, or extensive family or housing adjustments without first knowing what the client's physical and mental condition indicates.

The social worker is perhaps more aware than others concerned with the treatment of the cerebral palsied that the burden on the mother or caretaker may be very great. Exercises usually have to be performed at home, and many different ones may be prescribed by various specialists. The mother may find it impossible to do everything for the patient that is recommended. When too much is being asked of her, the social worker should encourage her to discuss her situation with the physician and physical therapist; in some cases, the social worker herself should point out to her professional colleagues what the home situation is like, and ask whether it is possible to treat the patient so as to make fewer demands on the mother.

CHARACTERISTIC FINANCIAL NEEDS

If the recipient needs therapy because of either cerebral palsy or its complications, transportation often presents a problem. Therapy is usually required for a long period; the recipient may not be able to use a common carrier, and he may need an attendant. Fortunately, private health agencies in many communities offer transportation service, or the social worker may be able to help the family secure it through volunteer services.

Other common needs include braces, crutches, wheel chairs, eyeglasses, hearing aids, specially built tables, ramps, bathroom rails, and a variety of other self-care devices ranging from walkers, to plastic bowls and tumblers set into trays, to elastic shoe laces. Nutrition is a frequent problem for the individual whose lack of control over upper extremities makes it difficult to get food into the mouth. Mealtime aids which lessen spillage may help materially.

All devices which provide support and stability or increase mobility, and which increase self-care and decrease family burdens, promote normality and harmonious relationships. These devices should be individually worked out with the advice of a therapist, nurse, or physician; often they can be homemade or created by a mechanically minded volunteer. Clothing may constitute a special financial problem, because it frequently needs adaptation to facilitate dressing and undressing and consequently cannot be easily secured at sales or through the second-hand clothing stores.

SPECIAL PROBLEMS WITH THE
SEVERELY HANDICAPPED

The possibility of institutionalization is a question which troubles the families of many severely handicapped recipients. If the family resolved the question in favor of keeping the invalid member at home during his childhood, it may arise again when the parents become elderly or too ill to provide the physical care necessary, or if they become concerned about what will happen to the invalid after their deaths.

This agonizing question may create such conflicts as to be immobilizing. The course of action which seems sensible and obvious to an outsider may be far from acceptable to the parents, because of the web of feelings in which they are caught. Sensitivity to the parents' feelings is necessary, as is the necessity of refraining from active participation in their decision unless the welfare of some other family member is being sacrificed to such a degree that counseling seems indispensable. Sometimes it helps to arrange for the family to visit the institution ahead of time, so that they can see for themselves what it is like.

If the family does decide to place the recipient in an institution, the members should be encouraged to visit him as often as possible even though it is painful. The patient deserves to know that he is still loved and has not been abandoned. The family can assuage their guilt over placing him when they know they are doing everything that is within reason to show him that they care. The family's transportation needs should be taken into account in financial planning.

Care by an attendant which will permit the caretaker to get away at regular intervals is often badly needed when the recipient remains at home. This may be less a budget problem than a counseling problem. The family may need help in finding a reliable person, and may also need help to overcome feelings of reluctance to let anyone else see the invalid or to trust him to anyone else's care.

If the recipient has frequent convulsions, it will be necessary to learn how recently he has been evaluated medically.

A physician can often prescribe medication which will make the recipient less difficult to handle, thus permitting an outsider to relieve the caretaker and at the same time reducing the caretaker's usual burden. If incontinence is an obstacle, more adequate supplies may lessen the caretaker's reluctance to let anyone else know how bad things are or increase the willingness of a sitter to stay with the recipient.

Some severely handicapped recipients who are shut-ins may be able to benefit from special group activities such as clubs which promote newspaper and correspondence activities and other indoor hobbies at home or in recreational centers.

RECREATION

Recreation is, for the severely handicapped as for others, a medium for personal growth and development. It offers socializing opportunities, teaches skills, dilutes self-interest and dependency, and is a constructive outlet for anxiety. Hobbies and social contacts serve as prevocational activities. As such, they deserve serious consideration both in the interview and in the budget plan.

The recreation and parks department of the city, the cerebral palsy associations, and Easter seals organizations provide opportunities for workers and parents to learn of available resources.

EDUCATION AND EMPLOYMENT

Although some educable cerebral palsied persons have little or no education, some with relatively normal or above normal intelligence are faced with the problem of overeducation in terms of employment. There seems to be an unhappy tendency on the part of counselors, parents, teachers, and others to foster a prolongation of the educational period of the cerebral palsied adult in order to delay the frustrating problem of securing employment.

He may be encouraged to think that he will be able to secure professional employment by virtue of advanced education when he does not have the physical qualities necessary or, in some instances, the emotional stability and maturity. Parents may have an unrealistic idea of what the child can accomplish, and the recipient may be quite unaware of the demands of the competitive world.

A disillusioning study made in New York[1] several years ago showed that more realistic vocational guidance is necessary in choice of scholastic pursuits, unless education is sought for its own legitimate civilizing function rather than as a vocational means. Of course we should not minimize the importance of the compensations of intellectual development for those physically handicapped persons whose intelligence permits the joys and escapes it provides.

Social workers are, with other counseling groups, tempted to misguide the eager, frustrated, intelligent cerebral palsied person into prolonged unsuitable schooling as vocational preparation rather than face, with the recipient and family, the painful realities of employer prejudices and physical requirements of various jobs.

Discouraging unrealistic vocational goals without damaging self-confidence requires much careful thought. Tact, kindness, and evidence of the worker's sincere respect for the recipient can mitigate the hurt which family or client feel when the worker cautiously questions unrealistic plans and leads them to consider the various requirements of the vocation under consideration. Exploratory interviews, in-

---

[1] Selma J. Glick, *Vocational, Educational, and Recreational Needs of the Cerebral Palsied Adult* (New York: Hunter College Chapter, International Council for Exceptional Children, 1953).

spection visits, and arrangements for aptitude testing and vocation counseling are some of the means which can be used to induce realistic thinking.

By and large, anything that induces self-consciousness or nervousness makes the medical condition less manageable, so that jobs which require public appearances or focus attention upon the person are unsuitable. Cosmetic, transportation, and speech requirements of the position as well as the physical strain and the amount of walking must be taken into account. Although special educational equipment does help greatly to compensate for lack of brawn in earning a living, caution should be exercised in choice of vocational goals to prevent later heartbreaks and bitterness.

The cerebral palsied person who attends school should be able to dress suitably and to have much the same things as the other students, such as lunch money and school supplies. Plans worked out with the rehabilitation agency should take into account these psychological needs, as well as transportation and physical problems posed by the disability, and by the architectural details of school buildings.

Attributes of personality may be more influential than the severity of disability in job finding and job holding, unless the patient is severely handicapped. The fact that the cerebral palsied person may have been greatly held back in socializing experiences, through delay in walking or talking or going to school, may retard his social maturity. Overprotecting parents may also create dependent, immature personalities in their cerebral palsied offspring. Any handicapped child who feels alone and different and friendless, especially during the painfully self-conscious period of adolescence, is likely to develop maladjustments which aggravate the problems of job finding and job holding.

Often the growing-up process is not accomplished until

a work experience provides the discipline, regularity, self-confidence, social contacts, and incentives that the recipient did not acquire at home or in school. Consequently, a period in a sheltered workshop or in a protected environment, such as a relative's business, social agency, clinic, or school, may serve as a transition to a better job and greater independence.

Sheltered employment may prove to be the only realistic vocational goal, because of the many handicaps of the cerebral palsied, and because of the strength of employer prejudice. Most important, sheltered employment is better than none.

FAMILY AND PSYCHOLOGICAL PROBLEMS

Crippling means different things to different people. A small disability can seem disastrous to one person, and a large one may be taken in stride by another. Much depends on what it meant to the parents to have a handicapped baby and how they treated the recipient in early childhood. Only as the worker begins to get some sense of what the condition has meant in the life of the particular family and the particular client can she successfully counsel a physically handicapped adult.

Dr. Earl R. Carlson, a specialist in cerebral palsy who himself is severely handicapped by the condition, has said that children of poor families grow up into more reliable, better-adjusted adults than those of well-to-do families because the parents could not afford to overprotect and shelter them excessively. Experience shows that families who place emphasis on intellectual attainment and social acceptability seem to have more difficulty loving a handicapped baby than people whose aims are not so directed. However, the parent-child relationship and the brother-sister relationship of a handicapped child differ in every family. Some poor families are just as ambitious and driving as some rich ones, and some are just as overindulgent.

The degree of insecurity and inferiority feelings of the recipient varies not only with the degree of true security he derived as a small child from the family relationships but with the actual physical frustrations and difficulties the disability caused and still causes. Prolonged physical dependence leads to emotional dependence. Deep mutual attachments of mother and child usually carry some resentful undertones, which may be either out in the open or quite unconscious.

Counseling—which may be a misnomer, because listening and encouraging usually play a much larger part than advice giving—must be directed toward something. It does not exist in a vacuum. The natural beginning is in regard to the client's budgetary needs, his relationship to the agency, and how he uses his assistance check. His medical supervision, vocational planning, and recreation follow as natural subjects around which the client-worker relationship is built.

Everything that encourages independence, self-respect, experience in handling money, and making decisions is growth producing. The client should not be told what to do or treated as if he were a child (unless he is so mentally retarded that this is necessary). If an overanxious or protective parent wants to do the talking or answer the worker's questions, it is always possible to indicate in a polite way that the worker would like to know the client's own reactions. Patience is necessary, particularly if the recipient's speech is impaired.

An objective but sympathetic worker who has demonstrated his genuine interest in the client will usually soon be drawn into the family's problems and relationships. The complaints, recriminations, bitterness, fantasies, unrealities, day dreams, distortions, burdens, as well as the extraordinary courage and selflessness and wisdom which various families and recipients demonstrate—all come out as the worker begins involving herself in ways to improve the recipient's self-care or vocational situation.

One reason why it is important to listen and move ahead slowly is that the client and his disability are inextricably interwoven with the rest of the family's situation and feelings. The burden of the recipient's disability sharpens and crystallizes conflicts and further weakens already weak places in the family fabric. Divorces, alcoholism, and other symptoms of strain seem to be prominent in families of cerebral palsied patients. Consequently, the complexity of the client's physical problem may be matched by the complexity of family relationships; even such seemingly trivial matters as the client's transportation to physiotherapy twice a week may have many ramifications.

The extent of the disability, though not the only determinant, is a major one. Families which could withstand the strain of a handicapped but ambulatory member may not be able to stand the cruel burden of a bedridden invalid. Not only is the mother involved, but the others who are deprived of the affection and strength she would normally put into their well-being.

Thus the worker may find herself the repository of many kinds of problems. Moral support, encouragement, and alleviation of burdens where possible are usually more helpful than aggressive counseling activities.

Teamwork with others is always time consuming, but several good resources for helping the recipient and family exist in most communities. The public health nurse is usually well acquainted with the problem of cerebral palsy through her work with crippled children; she will know of devices and resources and will have much to offer. The speech therapist, if there is one in the community, the occupational therapist, and the physical therapist have expert technical assistance to offer. If malnutrition is a problem, the home economist or nutritionist may be another valuable member of the team.

The physician should of course be the leader in dealing with the physical aspects of the client's care, and the vocational counselor in handling employment efforts. By having these persons help with the client's realistic daily problems and by coöperating with them over a period of time, the worker can help reduce some of the emotional problems of the recipient and his family. Renewed hope, knowledge of the interest and concern of others, and working toward goals which will mean greater satisfaction bring positive forces into play.

TERMS FREQUENTLY USED IN MEDICAL REPORTS

Abduction. The act of turning outward.

Adduction. The act of turning inward. *Abduction* and *adduction* are used to describe deformities or contractures—for example, "the foot is held in abduction" or "an adduction contracture."

Amentia. Congenital mental deficiency.

Anoxia. Lack of enough oxygen in the tissues to enable them to function properly. Marked lack of oxygen to the brain causes permanent serious results, such as mental retardation, cerebral palsy, paralysis.

Aphasia. Language disturbance caused by inability to comprehend, organize, or express thought.

Apraxia. Loss of ability to perform purposeful movements without paralysis of the parts concerned.

Arthrodesis. The surgical fixation of a joint or a permanent straightening. The operation is performed to provide stability.

Ataxia. Clumsiness and lack of balance.

Athetoid. Afflicted with slow, squirming, twisting, purposeless movements.

C.N.S. Central nervous system.

Chorea. An abnormal involuntary muscle activity, usually involving the arms and legs, of a quick jerky character.

Clonic. Pertaining to spasm in which rigidity and relaxation succeed each other.

Diplegia. Bilateral paralysis.

Extension. A movement which brings the members of a limb into or toward a straight condition.

Flexion. The act of bending or condition of being bent. Muscles are sometimes described as extensors or flexors.

Hamstrings. Tendons at the back of the knee.

Hemianopsia. Loss of half the visual field in one or both eyes.

Hypoxia. Low oxygen content. See *anoxia.*

Nystagmus. An involuntary, rapid movement of the eyeballs, sometimes described as a shimmering movement.

Osteotomy. Removal of part of a bone.

Scissors gait. A gait disturbance caused by the fact that spasticity of the muscles holds the thighs in adduction, causing the legs to draw together.

Spastic. Characterized by spasms.

Strabismus. Deviation of the eye which the patient cannot overcome; cross eyes.

Subluxation. An incomplete or partial dislocation.

Tendon, Achilles'. Heel tendon.

Tenotomy. The cutting of a tendon.

Tetraplegia. Paralysis of all four extremities.

CHAPTER X

Paraplegia and Quadriplegia

PERSONS WHO ARE PARALYZED below the waist are called *paraplegics*. Those who are paralyzed in all four extremities are called *quadriplegics*. Spinal cord injuries and poliomyelitis are the most common causes of paraplegia and quadriplegia. Other causes are spinal tumors and infections.

World War I first brought paraplegia and quadriplegia to general attention, but the early death of the victims avoided an accumulative problem. World War II again focused attention upon paraplegics and quadriplegics, and by this time modern medical measures were able to save their lives. Recurring poliomyelitis epidemics and the increasing number of automobile accidents added to the number of persons involved.

It is estimated that there are approximately 100,000 paraplegics and quadriplegics, including veterans, in the United States. The change in outlook within the past forty years, from death for all to complete rehabilitation for some, is so dramatic that the texts, particularly those from re-habilitation centers, tend to be overly optimistic. Although it is true that relative miracles can be performed in many cases, it is also true that the lives of most paraplegics are burdensome, frustrating, and physiologically complex. Suicide is the second largest cause of death among them. In order to be of greatest help, social workers need to be realistic as well as optimistic, and to understand what the patient must endure.

Young persons, especially men, are most liable to diving accidents and other accidents which produce cord injuries. Poliomyelitis is predominantly a disease of children and young adults. Therefore, paraplegics and quadriplegics are found among persons receiving assistance for aid to dependent children and aid to the disabled rather than in the old age assistance and aid to the blind caseloads. The severity and permanency of the handicap contraindicate general assistance except during the period of establishing eligibility and in supplementing categorical aid.

The problems caused by spinal cord injuries differ from those caused by poliomyelitis in many respects, but because paraplegia and quadriplegia, from whatever cause, have much in common, they are discussed together in this chapter.

General Medical Base for Social Planning

SPINAL CORD INJURIES

Physiology

The spinal cord, lying inside the protective bony spine, is a continuation of the nerve cells and bundles of the brain. Many pairs of nerves emerge attached to the cord by tiny roots. Voluntary muscle movements are relayed through the nerve cells in the cord. When the cord has "died" or atrophied below a certain spot where a fracture or wound has occurred, the limbs innervated by the nerve roots below the fracture can never move voluntarily again. Furthermore, the bowel and bladder cannot receive messages regarding control.

Muscle tone is also controlled by the nerve cells in the cord. Loss of normal tone results in either too great relaxation or too great contraction, so that painful spasm and rigidity or complete limpness can occur. The rigidity is described as *spastic,* and the limpness as *flaccid* paralysis.

If nerves have been injured but not destroyed, their power returns very slowly. How much they will be reactivated cannot be definitely determined for about eighteen months. However, a person with a spinal cord injury who is to regain some use of his muscles will usually begin to do so within a few months after the accident.

It is obvious that the level of the injury to the cord is, along with the extent, the determining factor in the physical disability. The higher the injury, the worse the effects. A broken neck or fracture of the *cervical spine* causes paralysis of the arms as well as the legs. If the injury occurs slightly lower, in the *thoracic* or *dorsal* spine, the person may have some arm movement. If the injury to the spine is at the waist or lower—a fracture of the *lumbar* or *sacral* spine—the upper part of the body will not be paralyzed.

COMPLICATIONS AND THEIR TREATMENT

The permanent paralysis of body and limbs results in secondary complications. These include poor circulation, which is conducive to pressure sores (*decubitus ulcers* or *decubiti*), a tendency to pneumonia, and especially to urinary infections (*pyelonephritis*), kidney stones (*renal calculi*), bowel impaction, and general debility. Now that antibiotics delay or prevent the early deaths that formerly occurred from infections, many clients can be restored to some measure of useful living in spite of their paralysis. This requires sufficient care to prevent bedsores, deformities, and recurring kidney stones and infections.

Bladder or kidney complications are among the most dangerous to life and the most difficult for the patient. Infections constitute the highest cause of death to paraplegics and quadriplegics. Depending on the site of the injury, most of the intelligent and well-motivated persons who are maintained in otherwise good health can be taught complete bladder control without use of a catheter; those who must wear catheters can, if intelligent, be taught unfailing control if they are provided with proper equipment and receive necessary help in weekly removal, cleaning, and sterilization of the catheter.

Thus, the incontinent patient who is not under medical care should always be referred to a physician to determine whether his injury is such that he could learn control if he had the opportunity.

Prevention of kidney stones is dependent in part on the patient's drinking substantial amounts of water; although this makes keeping dry more difficult, it is urged upon paraplegic patients. Prevention of stones is also dependent on the person's standing on his feet in his braces for about an hour a day; (this reduces the tendency for the minerals to leave the bones and make deposits in the kidneys). Someone must be available who has the time and inclination to help the patient into his braces; only the rare, athletic patient paralyzed below the waist can manage heavy, clumsy braces by himself.

Bowel training, said to be possible in more than 80 per cent of the cases, is accomplished by the use of suppositories and other methods until evacuation becomes possible by reflex at desired intervals. Bowel control requires strict adherence to a regulated diet to avoid a tendency either to impaction or to loose stools.

Pressure sores are further complications in all paraplegics, including those whose paralysis has been caused by polio-myelitis. Pressure sores are stubborn, difficult problems to overcome, and often require plastic surgery. These sores, like kidney stones, can be partly prevented if the patient stands in braces in an upright position. A bed patient must be turned every two hours; the wheel-chair patient must be taught to shift his weight frequently.

Constant vigilance is required by the patient and his family or caretaker in watching for red spots at likely pressure places, in avoiding binding or tight clothing, im-properly fitting shoes and brace straps, and in changing position often to remove pressure. Needless to say, lying on a lumpy mattress or sitting in a poorly fitting chair without a cushion is contraindicated, as is the use of hot water bottles or dangerous proximity to radiators. The patient cannot feel, and his safety lies in avoiding potential danger.

Contractures or deformities caused by improper posi-tioning in bed or chair and to lack of movement of the joints are best avoided by conditioning exercise performed on the patient regularly twice a day by someone who has been instructed by a physiotherapist. Bedding should be draped over frames designed to keep pressure off the feet, and the bed should be fitted with a footboard.

GENERAL CARE

Immediate hospitalization procedures after the injury are designed first to save the client's life, and later to prevent bedsores, deformities, and infections and to help the client develop such return of motion as may be possible. The most expert care obtainable should be secured, because the immediate care provided can determine whether the person can be rescued from permanent, complete paralysis.

Rehabilitation center treatment, although expensive, is worth while in helping the client learn as much self-care as possible, giving him a rehabilitation orientation and teaching him to use devices that reduce the burden his care will impose on the family. Institutional treatment frequently extends over many months, because complications often interrupt the course and retard the patient's recovery.

When the client returns home, supervision by a visiting nurse is essential, as is provision for continued medical supervision. The latter cannot be overemphasized. It is often thought that there is nothing further the doctor can do, because he cannot restore paralyzed limbs to usefulness. It is forgotten that care of the complications is of great importance to the patient's life and well-being.

POLIOMYELITIS

Only about 2 per cent of those who contract poliomyelitis are left with severe crippling. By no means should the disease be thought of as synonymous with paraplegia and quadriplegia, merely because it is a major cause of these conditions. The availability of Salk-type vaccine should eventually stamp out most new cases of poliomyelitis, but unfortunately lack of use of the vaccine, especially among the low-income group, makes this goal an indefinite one.

Poliomyelitis is predominantly a disease of young people, 80 per cent occurring in those less than eighteen years of age. However, in recent epidemics, adults have been attacked in large numbers. Stress of any kind (including childbirth, tonsillectomy, chilling or undue exertion) precipitates the disease. Poliomyelitis is caused by viruses spread from the nasal spray or excreta of carriers. The virus attacks the nerve cells in the spinal cord which control voluntary muscle movements. The cells that are killed will never regenerate; those that are only damaged may recover slowly up to eighteen months later.

Although the virus is likely to attack the cells controlling a regional set of muscles, it attacks them selectively rather than as a group or according to any certain level. Consequently, the muscle weakness may be patchy. A given extremity can have some strong muscles, some weak, and some entirely paralyzed.

Several consequences of this fact are of practical importance. Good muscles or tendons can be transplanted to take the place of the weak ones, thus widening the possibility that usefulness can be restored to limbs through treatment. Assistive devices can be tailored to the person to help compensate for loss of certain motions. The *orthotist* (device maker) is an especially important person in the care of poliomyelitis patients. Unfortunately, deformities are likely to be caused by the pull of good muscles against weak or useless ones. Physical therapy and bracing are therefore essential for minimizing the damage in many cases. An added gain from physical therapy is that the patient can be taught how to use the muscle strength he has, which can sometimes substitute functionally for what he has lost.

Because of the random muscle involvement and the fact that voluntary rather than involuntary muscles are attacked, there is not the permanent loss of bowel or bladder control in a paraplegic from poliomyelitis which occurs in the paraplegics from spinal cord injury. In the quadriplegic especially, however, there may be paralysis of the chest and diaphragm, and/or of the breathing and swallowing muscles, an even greater catastrophe than loss of bowel or bladder control.

Respiratory Impairments

An especially serious form of poliomyelitis, *bulbar polio-myelitis,* affects the swallowing mechanism and the muscles of the nose, throat, and face. Mortality is high during the early stage of this form of the disease.

Although the extent of paralysis and return of muscle function varies, the patient who retains some bulbar paralysis is an especially handicapped person. He is jeopardized by difficulty in eating and drinking. Common colds and pneumonia are hazardous to him; this fact has implications for nutrition and housing. The individual usually requires expensive suctioning equipment in the home and a person who has been taught to use it. He may have had a *tracheotomy* (an operation creating an opening into the windpipe) performed while acutely ill, and need to wear continuously a tracheotomy tube, which he must remove and cleanse or an attendant must do this for him.

Paralysis of the muscles used in breathing creates another form of respiratory problem. An "iron-lung" or tank type respirator is necessary for the patient with this form of paralysis. Living in a tank-type respirator is psychologically difficult and creates extra problems in physical care, so that patients are "weaned" to a partial respirator which fits over the chest, as soon as feasible.

An iron lung, a suction machine, and sometimes a rocking bed, another breathing aid, may be kept in the home of the severely involved quadriplegic or upper extremity paraplegic if he has respiratory problems. All this expensive equipment is usually provided by the National Foundation. The housing modifications necessary and the long-term arrangements for medical supervision and for the expense of an attendant (if someone other than a family member is required) are concerns of the family and the welfare department.

The Quadriplegic

Patients with paralysis of all four extremities as a consequence of poliomyelitis vary as to the nature and extent of crippling of each part. They may have enough motion in one arm to feed themselves or to write, or only incomplete paralysis in the trunk and legs so that they can move about to some extent. The particular physical condition of each person will determine his needs, problems, capacities, and outlook.

Quadriplegia is without peer as a catastrophe. Loss of use of the arms creates complete helplessness. Dependence on a chest respirator for breathing completes a picture of total physical dependence. Care at home is possible only under a combination of good family relationships and comprehensive planning. The patient can live indefinitely if he has good medical and nursing care.

Surprisingly enough, the patient is usually more comfortable at home than in an institution, once the difficult adjustment is made, because he eats better and his psychological needs are more adequately met. Great gain in use of impaired muscles is occasionally seen when the patient is highly motivated, even after the long convalescent period is over.

In the fortunately few cases where the patient has no motion below the neck, round-the-clock attention is required for prevention of bed sores, kidney infection, bowel impaction, and deformities, as well as for maintenance of life through attention to respiratory problems. This frequently includes care of a tracheotomy. If the home can be adapted for the patient's care, at least one skilled attendant is usually required for his care, in addition to a family member who has received some training at a hospital or rehabilitation center.

The Aftermath of Crippling

Frequently the public assistance agency's attention is drawn to a person who incurred severe crippling from poliomyelitis as a child or many years before application for aid. He perhaps made a good adjustment earlier, but now claims loss of strength and inability to perform the self-care or vocational activities formerly carried out. Question may arise as to whether the individual with a static condition really has deteriorated or whether he is malingering.

The question reveals the common fallacy of regarding loss of muscle strength as a static form of crippling. Overuse of weakened parts, or compensatory overuse of strong muscles, continued faulty positioning, imbalance in muscle pull, gain in weight owing to sedentary habits, the normal loss of muscle strength that occurs with aging, habitually poor diet, general weakening from illness, infection, or other stress—all combine to make muscle weakness into a slowly progressive rather than a genuinely static condition. The "old polio" requires continued, concerned medical supervision.

Implications for Public Assistance

THE EARLY STAGE

Profound psychological problems and family disruption inevitably occur when an active individual suddenly becomes a helpless person subject to lifelong frustration and discomfort. Great community expense is also inevitable because of the repeated hospitalizations and appliances the client must have, and because of the family support which is usually necessary. A long-time plan, carefully worked out from the beginning, and with the expenditures of time and money necessary to hold the family together and bring about some form of rehabilitation for the client, is the most economical course.

The suddenness of the catastrophe finds the patient and his family in the middle of every variety of human endeavors, problems, and relationships. "Unfinished business" (fortunately) distracts the patient and his family from the future, and often requires emergency financial assistance, child placement, homemaker service and other social measures. Sympathetic aid from neighbors, relatives, and officials often helps the family over the immediate emergency and during the early days of the disease or accident.

Unfortunately, after a few weeks or months, when the nature of the tragedy is completely appreciated by the patient and his family and discouragement settles over them, the extra efforts relatives and friends have made begin to pall. Thus, at the time of greatest need, the social worker must stand ready, because the organized resources of the community will often be required.

Prevention of eventual family disruption is the special province of the social worker. Other persons will be counseling and caring for the patient while he is hospitalized, but the worker is the person who must support the strength of the family. If the marriage partner is too self-centered and immature to weather a heavy burden, divorce or desertion will almost inevitably occur. If the spouse, on the other hand, has heroic strength, he may need but little help. However, with the average, ordinary spouse, who has some weaknesses and some strengths, the scales may well be tipped by needed help being given at the right time.

While the patient is still in the hospital or rehabilitation center, the spouse should be enabled to visit him frequently and to bring small things he needs. The spouse must have someone with whom to talk over his own problems. Babysitting services or transportation may be problems which should have thoughtful attention. Most of all, the spouse should not be pushed into a situation of having to earn the family's living and of taking care of the children at a sacrifice of time to visit the patient, or at the price of such fatigue that he sees the future through the dark haze of physical exhaustion.

THE RETURN HOME

A time of testing is the first week-end visit the patient makes to his home from the hospital or center. The responsibility of his care may place the spouse or caretaker in a panic; the patient may be unnerved at the revelation of the burden he is going to be on the loved ones. The social worker should be alert to the need for counseling soon after this first visit, giving the spouse the chance to get his fears out of his system, and thinking clearly with him about the different ways in which he can adjust things in order to manage. Moral support and realistic assistance to the family during these early days may save the marriage and keep the home together for the children.

The patient's discharge home usually requires a great deal of advance planning. It should be begun long before the patient is ready to leave the hospital. Provisions may be necessary for different housing, for the services of an attendant, and for household adjustments such as ramps or rails or widened doors. The patient may need a foam rubber mattress and seat cushion, wheel chair, braces, special clothing, orthopedic shoes, and perhaps even a suctioning machine. All these will have to be ready before he comes home.

The type of wheel chair for these patients is expensive, because it has to be especially tailored to the patient's bodily structure and needs. It should be the folding or portable kind which can be put in a car with him when he is taken to the doctor or goes to "school." It also must be equipped with brakes, for the chair must not roll while he is getting in and out of it. Service clubs can often be counted on to raise the money for a chair.

Service clubs may also pay for special devices. Many clever devices exist which increase self-care activities. If these cannot be secured locally, they can be obtained through the Fascole Corporation, 229 Fourth Avenue, New York 3, New York, which provides free catalogues on request. Needless to say, the patient's physician should approve the idea of the device before one is decided upon. Usually the hospital makes suggestions as to what is needed or desirable.

One of the most important measures is to secure, from the hospital social worker or physician and physiotherapist, an understanding of what the patient needs and what he can and cannot do for himself. An excellent description of the way in which the site of the injury affects the individual's life is found in an article in *Social Casework,* "Evaluating a Medical Symptom with Paraplegics," by two medical social workers in a Veterans' Administration hospital.* They describe the difference in functioning between two quadriplegics, one of whom has an injury at the fifth cervical vertebra and the other at the eighth. The first patient cannot lift a finger to help himself even to scratch his nose or to shoo away a fly; whereas the second can feed himself, hold his own cigarette, and shave with an electric razor. By contrast, a paraplegic who has good muscle power in his arms can learn to dress and undress

---

* Aaron Rosenblatt and Vincent W. Trovato, "Evaluating a Medical Symptom with Paraplegics," *Social Casework* XLI (March, 1960), 128–129.

himself and even to walk on crutches for short distances with the help of braces and crutches.

Every patient is different in what he can and cannot do for himself. This fact has myriad ramifications for social planning. It is not always easy to get this information, because hospital personnel are usually oriented to hospital life, not to care of the patient after discharge, and the social worker may need to be persistent. The biggest danger in rehabilitation is lack of correlation between phases of treatment by different agencies or institutions. Watch that the patient and his family do not fall between the cracks. A *Primer for Paraplegics and Quadriplegics** is an excellent source of information for family, patient, and worker about details of physical care.

Length of hospitalization is an area in which medical and social work personnel can often have rightful conflicts of interest. Rehabilitation center personnel, a singularly dedicated group, sometimes want to keep the patient until he can do everything they consider important, even though months may be required while the convalescing client slowly recovers from bedsores, fractures, kidney stones, and other complications. The social worker may need tactfully to keep them reminded of the gradual deterioration in family ties which take place when a member is away too long, and of the imperative nature of helping to keep the client's family together for his own good. If the client's hospitalization stretches over many months, the social worker should ask whether outpatient care would be satisfactory and, if so, attempt to work out the transportation and home care details with the help of hospital personnel and the patient's family.

---

* *Primer for Paraplegics and Quadriplegics* (New York: New York University-Bellevue Medical Center, 1957), Patient Publication No. 1.

Vocational rehabilitation agencies should be encouraged to supply their services in spite of the fact that limited, rather than full, self-support is all that the client can achieve. If the counselor seems slow or discouraged, special efforts should be made to stimulate interest, share information, and interpret needs. Some remarkable results have been achieved in limited vocational rehabilitation even with quadriplegics. However, quadriplegics require a great deal of the counselor's time. The social worker may need to be a constantly squeaking wheel, because the client may become too discouraged and immobilized to do much "squeaking" for himself.

Referral to vocational rehabilitation needs careful evaluation of the client's psychological readiness. Even though the outsider looking at the client accepts immediately that he is hopelessly crippled, he himself may not think of the condition as permanent. The shock of what has happened may be so great that he cannot absorb the truth. He may hold the idea that a miracle will happen, or cling desperately to falsely engendered hope, that he is going to recover.

We cannot destroy his faith or his hope without damaging his ultimate capacity to make the tremendous efforts that will be required of him to attain even a little capacity for self-care or self-support. If he does not openly object to vocational rehabilitation, but demonstrates lack of interest, he may either not yet be over the "grief" period, which sometimes lasts many months, or he may have given up all hope. Great tact, patience, and ingenuity are required of the physician, the caseworker, and the vocational counselor. Most important of all, the client must discover through experience that someone still believes in him and in his capacity to be a useful person.

Visiting nurse service is another "must" in these cases. Even though the client has been to a rehabilitation center and is now embarked on some form of rehabilitation, he still needs and will always need careful skin care and supervision of diet and activity. The public health nurse or visiting nurse should be encouraged to continue her interest in the case, even though the client seems uncoöperative. Most state health departments have medical social work consultants who can often be helpful in working with local nurses.

Incontinence is the most humiliating problem for the spinal cord injury patient. It is revolting to the spouse or caretaker, and causes an extra burden of laundry and care. As discussed earlier, most patients can be trained to bladder and bowel control. If the worker opens a case on a client who is incontinent or has only imperfect control, she should ascertain whether he can be sent to a hospital center to be trained. This matter may decide the vocational future and continuing family and social relationships, and is, consequently, well worth the continued necessary effort.

If the client cannot achieve bladder or bowel control, the necessary supplies must be provided, including two pairs of rubber pants, gauze padding, and two urinals (if the patient is male). Careful prescription of diet, habit regulation, fluid intake, and care of equipment, including catheter if used, are in the jurisdiction of the nurse and doctor. If, however, the worker finds that incontinence lies behind a client's seeming disinterest in vocational planning, or if she suspects it is partly responsible for his dependence and despair, she should secure medical and nursing consultation in order to determine whether the problem can be alleviated.

When the client is a man with a cord injury, marital problems caused by impotence may be very serious. These are frequently aggravated by the client's despair over not being able to support his family. Handling the assistance planning tactfully is important. It is highly important that the client be recognized as still the head of the family, so far as decisions are concerned. This means that such matters as the budget and the children's problems should be discussed with him, in spite of the necessity for home visits to do so.

It enhances the wife's and children's respect for the client (and his own self-respect) if they see that the agency thinks of him as a capable person, even if he is physically an invalid. It is often important that the wife be given plenty of opportunity to unburden privately to the worker, if she wants to, and that the client be given as much recognition and general emotional support as possible.

When the patient is a woman, housekeeper services on at least a part-time basis are essential in most cases. Such projects as lowering the kitchen shelves, and getting a low ironing board, for the client's use are usually economical in the long run. They also add to the client's morale, which is strengthened by her increased usefulness. If children are called upon to take on more responsibility than they should, they frequently leave home early. If the wife is allowed to languish in an institution, the husband often finds new interests. Consequently, holding the family together by means of a homemaker is often the most economical course as well as the kindest one.

SPECIAL PROBLEMS OF YOUNG ADULTS

Adolescence is a time of liberation from dependence on parents. Therefore nature causes the young person to resent dependence and to long to be his own self. Unfortunately, both poliomyelitis and spinal cord injuries frequently occur in late adolescence because of both recklessness and heightened physical activity at that time. The young married client who has barely succeeded in emancipating himself from the parental yoke and is just tasting the wine of independence is thus cast back into a dependent role. If he has an immature spouse who has deserted him, he must often go back under the parental roof; if she has remained loyal, he may have to go back and take her with him.

Conflict is compounded if liberation and youthful marriage generated some resentment and hurt in the parents. Having renounced their closeness to their child, the parents are now obliged to take him back and to change their way of life in order to care for a burdensome invalid.

It is apparent that family relationships may be extremely complex. A worker who remains sensitive to the meaning of words and actions of all concerned, not imposing nor prying, but manifesting concern and readiness to be helpful and discreet, may become a sounding board and a greatly needed source of strength.

TERMS FREQUENTLY USED IN MEDICAL REPORTS

Ambulate. To walk; usually referring to walking with braces or crutches.

Automatic bladder. A bladder trained to empty itself at regular intervals.

Bulbar poliomyelitis. An especially serious form of the disease in which there is disturbance of the swallowing mechanism and of the respiratory and circulatory systems.

C2, D5, L4, and so on. Describe the level of the injury. Refer to the number of the vertebrae and the section of the spine at which the injury took place. **C** stands for *cervical;* **T** for *thoracic,* which is another name for *dorsal;* **D** for *dorsal;* **L** for *lumbar;* **S** for *sacral. Cervical,* or neck, is the highest section, consequently the most serious to injure; dorsal (or *thoracic*) *next;* then *lumbar;* then *sacral.*

Cystoscopy, retrograde pyelogram, urogram. Common names for kidney tests; the latter two refer to dye injection followed by X ray.

Cystostomy. An operation in which a small opening is made into the bladder either to remove large kidney stones or in some instances to insert a catheter.

Cystotomy. The operation of making an incision into the bladder.

Decubiti. The plural of *decubitus ulcers;* bedsores.

Flexion contracture. A deformity in which the limb is bent or contracted at the joint.

Gantrisin. A sulfa drug frequently used for kidney infections.

Kyphosis. Humpback, an abnormal curvature of the spine.

Laminectomy. Surgery to remove some of the bone at the back of the vertebrae, frequently performed early in spinal cord injury cases to ascertain the extent of the actual damage to the cord and to relieve pressure on it.

Laminectomy with spinal fusion. Laminectomy followed by grafting bone on the place weakened by the laminectomy.

Lordosis. A curvature of the spine with the opposite effect of kyphosis; the convexity is forward.

Micturition. The act of emptying the bladder.

Myelo. The Greek root pertaining to the spinal cord.

Myelogram. Test to determine the place of the injury, performed by injecting a dye into the cord and then taking an X ray.

Myelopathy. Pathology of the cord.

Osteotomy. The surgical cutting of a bone.

Paresis. Partial paralysis; sometimes loosely used to describe *paraplegia.*

Plegia. The term for paralysis; *quadriplegia,* four extremities paralyzed; *paraplegia,* the two lower extremities paralyzed. *Hemiplegia* refers to one half of the body, but this occurs in strokes, not from spinal cord injury.

Renal. Pertaining to the kidneys.

Renal calculi. Kidney stones, to which the cord injured are subject.

Rhizotomy. Surgery to cut nerve roots causing intractable spasms.

Scoliosis. Abnormal curvature of the spine; one of the fairly common deformities caused by poliomyelitis.

Sphincters. Muscular valves located at mouth of bladder and rectum; technically, a muscle closing any natural orifice.

Spinal paralytic poliomyelitis. The common form of the disease.

Tenotomy. Cutting of a tendon.

Tidal drainage. A method used in hospitals to train persons with denervated bladders to regain inhibitory control so that incontinence is overcome without the use of a catheter.

Tracheotomy. Formation of an artificial opening into the trachea, or windpipe.

Transverse myelopathy or transected cord. A severing or crushing of the cord; causes permanent paralysis below the level of the severance.

CHAPTER XI

Cardiovascular Disease and Diseases of the Outlying Vessels

HEART DISEASE far outranks all other diseases in causing death and disability. It occurs among all ages, and is of several kinds. Social factors may literally play a life-and-death role in its treatment. Consequently, social workers have an unusual opportunity to help in preventing invalidism, family disruption, and death from this most common of all chronic illnesses.

Because the heart is but one part of the circulatory system, inseparable in operation from the blood vessels, heart disease is termed *cardiovascular disease* (C.V.D.).

A more comprehensive name, which takes cognizance of the close relationship of the heart and blood vessels to the kidneys, is *cardiovascular renal disease*.

Of the many kinds of heart disease, the most common now is *coronary* disease (*arteriosclerotic heart disease* or ASHD). More men than women have this condition, especially those less than fifty years of age. The incidence in both sexes, however, grows greater in later years. The other two most common forms are heart trouble due to high blood pressure, *hypertensive cardiovascular disease* (HCVD) and *valvular heart disease.* All three, if sudden death does not intervene, terminate in *congestive heart failure,* which is a specific disease entity referring to a heart so weak that it cannot pump the blood out fast enough and congestion therefore occurs.

Heart disease in children will not be described, although it should be remembered that rheumatic fever in childhood often causes valvular disease in adult life, which is one of the reasons that the social problems in children with rheumatic fever need such careful attention.

Two considerations should be taken into account in our thinking about heart trouble. The first is that excessive fear and sometimes unnecessary invalidism characterized it in the era just past, and that there is a pendulum swing at the present time to false cheeriness in much of the literature put out for common consumption. We need to take some of the optimism with a grain of salt.

The other consideration is the imperfect incorporation of psychosomatic concepts in medical practice and the medical fringe groups. Professional persons have become so conscious of the place of anxiety in causing physical aberrations that we often jump quickly to the false conclusion that something is "psychosomatic," or, derogatorily, that it is "neurotic." The symptoms of heart disease—especially of the most common type, coronary trouble—cannot be objectively confirmed in many instances, in the manner in which for example an X ray confirms tuberculosis. Further, the individual usually looks well.

Consequently, we are sometimes guilty in public assistance of considering certain seriously ill clients as complainers or lazy and unwilling to work if a superficial physical examination has minimized the disability. Placement in occupations that are too strenuous occasionally seems to be made by collaborating rehabilitation agencies. Because exertion and strain are of critical importance in the client's life, extra caution is necessary in the evaluation of and planning with clients with this disease.

General Medical Base for Social Planning

PHYSIOLOGY

The social worker needs to understand medical reports and doctors' statements, which often do not make sense unless he understands the circulatory system. Consequently, owing to the frequency of heart disease in all caseloads, it is worth the worker's time to try to acquaint herself with the circulatory background and the terms used.

The Circulation

As is well known, no tissue can live which does not receive oxygen and a constant supply of other nutrients. These are brought to the organs by the blood vessels, and the heart is the pump which gets the blood there.

The heart is a two-sided pulsating hollow chamber. Each of the separate sides has two parts connected by valves. The lower parts which do the pumping are called *ventricles;* the upper parts which are collecting stations are called *auricles*. A large blood vessel, the *aorta,* is connected by a valve to the left ventricle; another large artery, the *pulmonary artery,* is connected to the right ventricle. The left ventricle pumps the fresh, nutrient blood into the aorta and from there out into the smaller arteries throughout the body. When the arteries reach their terminal points they connect with or become veins, which bring the blood back minus its oxygen and food, having picked up carbon dioxide and other impurities. This impure blood flows into the right heart, which sends it into the lungs for oxygen refreshment. From there it goes into the upper part of the left heart, is pumped down through the valve into the left auricle, and then starts all over again.

In order to fit the heart muscle for such heavy work, its own blood supply has been provided by a separate set of arteries. Because they fit over the top of the heart like a crown, they are called the *coronary* arteries. When one of these becomes blocked or damaged, the heart muscle does not get a sufficient supply of blood, causing heart damage which will be described later.

The Heart Beat

The actual beat or rhythm of the heart stems from the brain via electrical impulses from a nerve. The impulses spread over the heart in a certain pattern, which can be traced by the electrocardiograph (ECG or EKG). The tracing that is made is an *electrocardiogram;* the machine that makes it, the *electrocardiograph.* When the rhythm changes from normal, either because the heart is damaged or because there is a physiological disturbance in the body, an *arrhythmia* is said to exist.

The arrhythmias may be relatively meaningless or they may be very serious, depending on what they are and what are the other physical signs of cardiac disturbance. Slow rhythm is called *bradycardia;* fast rhythm, *tachycardia;* most significant, irregular rhythm, *fibrillation.* The social worker should know that these words are not diagnoses but names of physical symptoms or findings, that they may have complicating significance which should be ascertained from the doctor.

The EKG is so common a test that any good examination for heart disease includes one or more. This measurement of electrical impulses always confirms substantial damage from valvular disease but does not always measure coronary or hypertensive disease. There is some tendency to believe that if the EKG is normal, there is nothing wrong with the patient. Unfortunately, the test is not so comprehensively accurate as to make this true.

The Kidneys, Liver, and Brain

The kidneys, like the lungs, are an inseparable part of the circulatory system because they too filter away impurities in the blood. In addition, they provide the mechanism for maintaining the fluid balance in the body as well as the balance of certain chemicals; among other things, they adjust the amount of water and salt excreted. In order to do their very complicated work, they must have a certain blood pressure and an adequate blood supply. Their interdependence with the heart is the reason why a urinalysis is part of the laboratory work essential in a heart examination.

High blood pressure, when it lasts long enough, damages the kidneys; conversely, kidney disease can elevate the blood pressure. As kidney (*renal*) tissue cannot be restored, the patient's outlook is gravely affected when there are signs that it has been damaged.

The liver is also closely involved with the heart, because among its other functions it stores blood which is not in use and partly regulates blood volume. When the heart becomes congested because of disease, the liver becomes full and congested too. Consequently, the size of the liver is one of the important diagnostic signs in advanced heart disease. On medical reports the size is usually noted by the number of fingerbreadths the doctor can feel it below the ribs—for example, "liver down 2fb." Or the report may simply note hepatomegaly ("hepato" meaning "liver," plus "megaly" meaning "abnormally large"). Like kidney damage, liver damage is a sign of permanent serious complications.

The brain has first call on the blood supply, which arrives via an artery branching off the aorta. It is supplied locally by myriads of tiny blood vessels that carry oxygen to all its tissues.

Extra Demands upon the Heart

Any part of the body, including the stomach, which is being exercised needs more blood. When a person is cold, his outlying vessels become constricted by nerve action, causing the heart to work harder to get the blood in. Thus, it can be seen why calls on the heart for more blood from several places at once are likely to "embarrass" it, or why an extra call from even one place can embarrass a weakened heart or one fed by a faulty circulatory system. These facts explain why there are more heart attacks after meals, more cardiac deaths in winter, and why medical recommendations forbid heavy exercise, walking in the cold wind, suggest several light meals rather than three heavy ones, and so on.

An additional source of demand for greater cardiac output is anxiety or strong emotion. When the brain receives signals from the senses that danger is in sight, psychologically or in reality, it uses the master gland (pituitary) to ready the body physiologically for action. We have all experienced the way the heart leaps into action in response to hormonal stimulation.

This survival technique of the body can be unfortunate. The patient with a damaged heart may fall dead from the heart's inability to meet the demand for swiftly expanded action. Conversely, the individual with little organically wrong with his heart may put such a strain on it through anxiety that the circulatory mechanism is thrown out of balance, creating physical symptoms of circulatory imbalance that further frighten the patient and confuse the doctor.

This interchange of psychic and physical stimuli (a good illustration of the psychosomatic concept) suggests why reassurance is helpful to heart patients, and also why the individual who does have symptoms but is told that there is nothing wrong with him grows all the more anxious.

The Blood and Blood Vessels

The blood and the blood vessels themselves have an important part to play in heart trouble. Blood is made up of a fluid (*plasma*) in which various cells are suspended, and the food, oxygen, hormones, and waste products it transports to their destinations. The fluid, which is largely water, is described as clear except after meals, when it becomes milky looking from the small globules of fat suspended in it. In addition to the materials and cells it transports, the plasma contains proteins and mineral salts.

The salts and proteins are important in maintaining the proper balance between the water in the tissues and in the blood. When the water seeps out of the blood stream, owing to a variety of reasons in heart and kidney dysfunctions, and waterlogs the tissues, *edema* is said to exist. *Pedal edema* occurs if the waterlogging is at the ankles; *pulmonary edema,* if in the lungs; and *ascites,* if the fluid has collected in the abdomen.

The vessels themselves are supple muscular pipes ranging in size from the large aorta to minuscule peripheral or outlying vessels. Their gradual hardening in later life is part of the aging process, but can develop at any age for pathological reasons. The cholesterol from the fats carried in the blood stream attaches itself in little plaques to the inner walls and accumulates like rust in water pipes. This condition is called *atherosclerosis*. Whereas the process is often widespread throughout the arteries, it may exist only in patches—for example, in the coronary vessels or in those of the legs or the brain.

When the vessels become hardened and thickened inside, the blood has to push harder to get through, which raises the blood pressure, and this, in turn, gradually damages the vessels. The relationship between high blood pressure and hardening of the arteries is a two-way affair, as either can cause or aggravate the other. This does not mean, of course, that high blood pressure is always caused by hardening of the arteries. Hypertension as a disease will be discussed later.

Blood pressure readings refer to the amount of blood pushed out by the heart when it contracts and when it is resting between contractions. The above-the-line reading is the *systolic* or contracting pressure, and the below-the-line reading is the *diastolic* or resting pressure. An important thing for social workers to remember in reading medical charts is that it is the pressure reading below the line, not the one above the line, which is of greatest importance in indicating pathology. The below-the-line pressure is considered normal up to a maximum of about 90. It is also important to realize that one reading is not too significant, because blood pressure varies with posture and nervous tension.

MAJOR FORMS OF HEART DISEASE

The different kinds of heart disease affect the body in different ways. Each has its own set of symptoms and treatment, and a different set of terms are encountered. The discussion which follows separates each major form of the disease and includes a section on diseases of the outlying vessels. The reader who is interested in learning about a specific form of the disease in connection with a given case may select the topic he is interested in and omit the remainder of the medical discussion. It is suggested, however, that the first section on cardiac decompensation be included, because any form of heart disease can end in or be mixed with this condition.

Cardiac Decompensation

The eventual outcome of all forms of heart disease, if sudden death has been avoided, is *congestive heart failure*. This is a term used to describe the condition in which a weakened heart cannot get enough blood to the tissues and in which excess blood accumulates in certain organs. The patient experiences shortness of breath (*dyspnea*) on slight exertion; fluid accumulates in his ankles (*pedal edema*) and in his lungs (*pulmonary edema*). The doctor can hear the fluid in the lungs by listening; describes the sound as *rales*. The patient is frequently unable to sleep lying flat; he has sudden attacks of shortness of breath at night; the rhythm of his heart is disturbed; and he is sometimes in severe pain.

Cardiac failure (sometimes called *decompensation*) constitutes an emergency. The client must have immediate medical treatment, usually in a hospital. The administration of digitalis or one of its derivatives will often stimulate the heart enough so that it can do its work relatively well over a long period. The diet must be restricted in salt and other forms of sodium to discourage retention of fluid or waterlogging in the organs. Weight reduction may be necessary; sometimes diuretics or kidney stimulants are given by injection; and physical and mental rest is required.

Unless the heart is too badly damaged, it will compensate or adjust to this modified demand and the symptoms will largely disappear. The client who is enabled by good medical treatment, environmental manipulation, and counseling to follow the doctor's recommendations strictly may live several years. Even though his state is precarious and his physical activity and diet are greatly restricted, he can still contribute to the supervision and well-being of his family.

High Blood Pressure

When blood pressure readings are consistently high, the individual is said to have hypertension. Some hypertension is caused by kidney disease, but most of it is of unknown origin and is referred to as *essential hypertension*. Unless death intervenes, it always progresses to the point where heart, vessels, kidneys, and brain are affected, at which time it is called *hypertensive cardiovascular disease*.

In most cases the progression is very slow and the individual has no symptoms or only slight ones for many years. This is called *benign* hypertension. In a relatively small number of patients, the course of the disease is extremely rapid, and the disease is characterized as *malignant* or *accelerated* hypertension. Malignancy or acceleration usually occurs from the beginning, with death occurring within a few months or a year, but it can develop suddenly in an individual who has had benign hypertension for a long time.

For a person with high blood pressure a comprehensive examination includes the eyes to determine whether the vessels have become damaged, as indicated by the condition of the small arteries behind the eyeball. Examination includes also X ray of the chest to determine whether the heart has become enlarged as a result of extra work; the urine is analyzed to find out whether the kidneys have become affected. Personality changes, if any, are also noted, because these may show that the blood vessels to the brain have become affected. If none of these things have shown up, and if the individual stays on medication and the proper regime, his health can remain good for years.

Because the cause of hypertension is unknown, its treatment is not specific until there is concrete evidence of damage to the organs and vessels, except that weight reduction is considered important, when indicated, as is avoidance of anxiety and excesses of all kinds. Since there is a possible emotional component in high blood pressure, it is considered important, medically as well as humanely, that the patient not be made anxious over his condition.

Whether or not the actual level of the blood pressure has anything to do with the progression of the disease is evidently a moot medical point. However, it seems to be accepted medical practice to try to lower the pressure by drugs, diet, and calm. It seems logical that the less the pressure, the less quickly damage will occur to the organs and vessels.

Since there is doubt as to the importance of the actual level of pressure, the social worker should not jump to conclusions from looking at the blood pressure readings alone. However, when there is a below-the-line pressure of ninety or higher, it is worth finding out from the physician whether there are signs of damage to the vessels, heart, kidneys, as these indicate complications which in turn indicate severe disease.

Hypertension is one of the cardiovascular problems which have sometimes been dramatically treated by surgery. The operation is on the sympathetic nerves rather than on the heart. By no means are all patients good candidates for the operation, and worth-while results are said to have been obtained only in a small number but in this group the relief has been outstanding. When possible, clients who have been suggested by their doctors for this operation should be sent to a teaching center. Postoperative disability is said to last for at least six months and often longer.

Brain damage from high blood pressure is unfortunately one of its common manifestations. This ranges from forgetfulness, irritability, inability to concentrate, headaches, giddiness, and feeling of falling forward, to blackouts, convulsions, and strokes caused by severe pressure, and finally hemorrhage of a blood vessel in the brain or by a blood clot in one of the arteries. Alleviation of this kind of distress and prevention of cerebrovascular accidents are, of course, two of the reasons for obtaining regular medical supervision, with provision of antihypertensive drugs and a suitable regime.

When the heart becomes damaged by hypertension, it becomes enlarged and eventually unable to keep up with demands. The symptoms and the treatment become those of congestive failure, previously described.

Arteriosclerotic Heart Disease

It will be remembered that arteriosclerosis refers to hardening of the arteries, an inevitable concomitant of advancing age; that atherosclerosis refers to "rusting of the pipes," or the deposition of fatty substances in the arteries which turn to calcium and, therefore, harden and narrow the channels; consequently, the terms are not synonymous, but the conditions are closely related. Arteriosclerotic heart disease is sometimes referred to as atherosclerotic heart disease. The term *coronary disease* is also used for approximately the same condition, referring to hardening and thickening of the vessels that nourish the heart muscle itself.

It will also be recalled that atherosclerosis can occur diffusely throughout all the vessels or only in spots. There is no way to measure it objectively, which is unfortunate, because this form of heart disease is the most common, accounting for more than half of the deaths. People can have hypertensive and arteriosclerotic heart disease at the same time because of the close relationship between hypertension and hardening of the arteries.

For our purposes, coronary trouble (ASHD) is primarily of two kinds. The channels of the coronary arteries may be so narrowed and filled up with fatty or calcified patches that the blood has difficulty getting through, especially when emotion or exertion make calls on the heart for extra work. This is referred to as *myocardial ischemia,* which means that the heart muscle is starving for blood because of the disparity in supply and demand. It causes pain in the left chest, shoulder and arm and, though transitory, can be extremely severe. The disease is commonly known as *angina pectoris* ("angina" meaning "pain" and "pectoris" "of the chest").

The course of the disease may be interrupted by sudden death, or it may progress at an uncertain pace until an important vessel is completely closed, when the person dies because of complete starvation of blood to the heart muscle. Some persons live for many years with this condition and die of another cause entirely, but their prognosis is uncertain.

The other and better-known course of coronary disease is as follows: an ulceration occurs at the site of a plaque and a clot forms, blocking the vessel. This is called a *thrombosis.* More rarely, a piece of hardened material is sloughed off the side of a vessel and is transported to a narrow spot, where it blocks the flow of blood to the heart. The piece of material is called an *embolism* or a clot. It *occludes* the vessel—a coronary occlusion.

The part of the heart muscle that was nourished by this artery dies—referred to as *infarction* or death of that part. The person has had a "heart attack," or a *coronary occlusion,* or a *coronary embolism,* or a *myocardial infarction*— all meaning the same thing. There may have been no warning at all, or the person may have had the pain from ischemia for some time.

From two-thirds to three-fourths of the persons who have infarctions survive. The first two to four weeks are critical, and the individual must be provided with hospital care and skilled treatment. Some make a good recovery within six months, and are able to proceed, though with caution, with a modified normal life, especially if they are accustomed to sedentary occupation and are in circumstances which permit enough rest, proper diet, and mental calm. Others, especially those who have had large infarctions, develop complications, have serious symptoms, and are invalids until death.

The aftermath of myocardial infarction is variable. At best it is apparent that the person who has recovered after a six-month period has two problems to live with the rest of his life. A piece of his heart muscle is dead, and the heart's total capacity is, therefore, permanently weakened. Another problem is that the atherosclerotic blood vessel which sloughed off one clot may slough off another one at any time.

Treatment is based on recommendations for less work for the damaged heart: low-salt and reducing diets, avoidance of worry and exertion (especially lifting), avoidance of cold and of large meals. Further, a low-fat diet is usually recommended with the hope of slowing down the atherosclerotic process. Tobacco is usually forbidden, and often a blood-thinning or anticlotting drug is given. The latter requires close laboratory supervision because it is potentially hazardous.

Valvular Heart Disease

It will be recalled that the pumping chambers or ventricles of the heart are connected with the collecting stations or auricles by valves, and also that the left ventricle opens into the large blood vessel (the aorta) by means of a valve. These valves are like trap doors that open and shut to let the proper amount of blood through at the right moment.

The streptococcal infection which causes rheumatic fever has a proclivity to infect the valves. The resultant scar tissue "rusts the hinges of the doors." The valves are specified as *mitral* and *aortic*. The stiffening of the valves is called *stenosis*. If not enough blood gets in, insufficiency is said to result; if it flows back where it does not belong, *regurgitation* is the term used.

Hence, one finds, especially in former rheumatic fever patients, mitral stenosis and/or aortic stenosis, sometimes with regurgitation and/or insufficiency. These conditions have different implications medically and a wide variation of degrees, symptoms, and complications. The most common form is mitral stenosis. In both mitral and aortic disease, the onset may be gradual, with no outstanding symptoms except fatigue and malaise. The diagnosis is, therefore, difficult in the early stages, and the patient may be considered a hypochondriac or malingerer.

Of particular interest to social workers are several factors, among them being the fact that certain selected uncomplicated patients with mitral stenosis are candidates for one of the remarkable heart operations, *mitral commissurotomy*.

The risk of the surgery depends not only on the skill of the surgeons and the facilities of the hospital but on the proper medical selection of the candidates. All clients who have mitral valve disease deserve the chance to go to a large medical center (where the interest in the client for teaching purposes should ensure free care) to see whether they are good candidates for the operation. They should never be urged to have the surgery, because it is a major risk and does not guarantee cure.

If the patient cannot be helped by surgery or if he has had valvular disease for a long period before it is performed, the heart muscle stretches out of shape as a result of its heavy burden in trying to do its work with inefficient valves. Like a rubber band which has been stretched too far, it loses its elasticity or, in other words, its capacity to respond to sudden or extra demands. One of the diagnostic signs of a damaged heart is enlargement (*cardiac hypertrophy*).

It is a life-or-death matter for a person with a stretched, inelastic heart and inefficient valves to live within his cardiac reserve. If he does, barring complications, he can get along well for a long time; if he does not, he may fall dead or go into cardiac failure. That is why the doctor so often tells the patient to "take it easy." Unless this innocuous-sounding recommendation is translated into practical terms and the importance understood by client and social worker, it is likely to be meaningless.

Valvular disease is usually found in young or middle-aged adults—the mothers of young children and the wage earners. The practical reorganization of family life and occupations may, therefore, become the most important single factor in preventing death or invalidism. Further pregnancies for the woman are frequently contraindicated, which creates an entire train of complications, especially in some families.

Diseases of the Outlying Vessels

The outlying or peripheral blood vessels are subject to several pathological conditions; not all these conditions are circulatory, but because atherosclerosis is the most common of them, diseases of the peripheral vessels are most conveniently mentioned in connection with cardiovascular disease. The term used for the broad grouping is *peripheral vascular disease* (P.V.D.).

When the vessels of the lower legs start filling up with "rust," as happens especially in older men, and the blood flow with oxygen nourishment to the tissues is reduced, the patient's feet are cold, his toes feel numb, his skin looks shiny and discolored and is subject to ulceration. He may become completely disabled for anything but sedentary work because the exercise of walking, even a short distance, causes such cramps in his calves that he cannot go on. The condition is called *intermittent claudication*.

There is no treatment except for hope of slowing down the process by a low-fat diet. Other than the diet, the most important aspect of care is prophylactic care of the feet. This means careful attention to corns and bunions, avoiding cold and chilling, keeping the feet scrupulously clean, having well-fitting socks and shoes with no holes, bulky harsh darns, or areas of irritation. If blisters or sores develop, there is great danger of gangrene because of the precarious state of the poorly nourished tissues.

Peripheral ischemia (blood starvation in the extremities) can also be caused by *thromboangiitis obliterans,* or *Buerger's disease*. It is an inflammatory process of unknown origin occurring mostly in young men. This painful disease progresses at a variable pace, frequently resulting in the amputation first of one and then another extremity and creating, of course, great anxiety and progressive disablement.

The pace of the disease is said to slacken off in from ten to twelve years. Symptoms and treatment are generally similar to those of atherosclerosis of the extremities, with the exception that there is extreme emphasis upon not smoking because smoking constricts the arteries and apparently extends the progression of the disease. Giving up smoking is a special problem in Buerger's disease, because of the pain and sleeplessness the disease causes.

The disease is difficult to diagnose in its early stages and, therefore, it is important for social workers to guard against assuming that the client's complaints are hypochondriacal. Expert medical care is required. Great damage can be done by hasty or inefficient medical practice or by quackery.

Occasionally social workers have clients with *Raynaud's disease,* another peripheral vascular condition of unknown origin. This condition is different from those previously described in that it is caused by spasm of the digital (fingers and toes) arteries, is mostly a disease of high-strung, underweight women. In mild form the disease is merely a nuisance, especially during the winter, but in severe cases it progresses to the point where great pain and amputation results.

More common in our caseloads are *thrombophlebitis* and *varicose veins,* both diseases of the veins rather than of the arteries. *Thrombophlebitis* is ordinarily thought of as an acute condition following surgery or childbirth, requiring rest in bed, and dangerous chiefly because of the possibility of a clot passing to the lung. However, repeated attacks with prolonged impairment of the circulation in the affected leg cause chronic swelling, ulceration, and pain which is permanent and very disabling because of the individual's inability to be on his feet.

Varicose veins are another condition usually considered relatively minor and amenable to conservative measures such as elastic stockings and elevation of the leg, or to injections or surgical removal of the affected veins. The condition becomes a matter for serious concern when repeated attempts at treatment prove unsuccessful and the deep circulation of the leg is permanently impaired. In these cases the classical symptoms of edema (swelling) pain, and discoloration and ulceration of the skin (so-called *trophic changes*) cause permanent disability for all but sedentary occupations.

Implications for Public Assistance

MEDICAL QUESTIONS

When a formerly self-supporting individual applies for public assistance because heart disease has stopped his employment, or when a client develops heart disease, the caseworker asks herself three questions. For what type of aid is he eligible? Can he be rehabilitated? What can the agency do to prolong his life and minimize his disability?

Access to a good medical report and then to a fruitful conference with the physician are the first steps in answering all three questions. Reports can often be secured from the physician who has been treating the client; otherwise, the best possible physical examination needs to be arranged. Equipped with the report and having looked it over carefully, the worker will decide what questions she needs to ask the physician to secure an estimate of the client's present physical condition and the regime he should have.

She can make sure at the same time that the client has received adequate interpretation of his condition. Ordinarily we think of the client as our best source of information. This is not true regarding illness, especially serious, worrisome illness, as was brought out in Chapter I. The physician often deliberately minimizes the seriousness of heart trouble in talking to the client. However, he should make sure his recommendations are clear, and that the client knows that they are important to act upon. The worker often finds that this has not been accomplished. Because she is bound by professional ethics to keep the physician's confidence, and is not equipped to give interpretations herself, she should refer the client and his family to the doctor for a further discussion of medical recommendations.

That the client's impairment is permanent is obvious

from the diagnosis. Whether his current condition can be expected to improve somewhat, at least temporarily, will depend on the kind of disease he has, how long he has had it, how severe the damage is, how he has responded to treatment, and whether a suitable social situation can be achieved.

For example, in mitral stenosis, the worker will need to find out from the doctor whether the client may be considered a candidate for evaluation of the possibility of surgery. In any kind of valvular disease she will want to know whether the heart is compensated or in failure, and if the latter, whether this condition is acute and expected to respond to treatment or whether it is chronic and resistive to treatment. If the client has had his first myocardial infarction and it is of recent date, the worker will know that rehabilitation may be a possibility later, but that, meanwhile, a continuing assistance grant is justified and that every effort needs to be made toward a maximum of protection and minimum of strain.

A client who has shortness of breath or pain on mild exertion, with the physical findings that usually accompany these symptoms, and who has had the advantage of good treatment without response, is a suitable applicant for aid to dependent children, aid to the disabled, or for OASDI. In other words, it is probable that he is totally as well as permanently disabled, and the agency's goal will be to make the client as secure, cheerful, and comfortable as possible.

The application process is not separate from the social treatment. The client should be treated like a responsible individual and should not be given the impression that he is expected to fall dead; at the same time there is the need to minimize exertion and anxiety-producing features of the application process in every possible way.

The earlier discussion of physiology attempted to make clear that heart disease is one in which a direct relationship exists between social treatment and the well-being and longevity of the client. Whereas many other factors, some related to pathology and some to the adequacy of medical care, also determine life or death, the patient's adaptation of activity and environment to his condition is essential.

OCCUPATION

Suitable occupation is important whatever the client's condition. The occupational goal may be merely therapy or it may be return to self-support, depending upon the client's physical condition, his vocational background, and how much the doctor thinks it is safe for him to do. Life is cruel when burdened by the constant fear of sudden death or of the agony of an attack. Unless the client has something to occupy his mind, morbid fears and anxiety will take over, which in themselves add burdens upon the heart.

Further, enough exercise to keep the circulation in good order and the body working naturally is medically indicated, except during certain periods of treatment or at the terminal stage of illness. Regular, planned exercise on an individualized basis has in fact come to be considered an important part of treatment, not for all heart patients, but for the large group of cardiacs who have had a myocardial infarction and who have made a good recovery. The most natural way to get exercise is in connection with work.

The problem of the cardiac housewife and mother of children is, of course, how to cut down on work. She faces severe problems of self-discipline and adaptations. She is most frequently a patient with valvular (rather than coronary) disease, who must not exert beyond the capacity of her heart and who has been advised to discontinue effort before the fatigue point is reached. The details of her responsibilities, with the amount of effort involved in each, should be discussed with her and with the physician. Washing, ironing, scrubbing, washing windows, woodwork, and walls, carrying groceries from the store or into the house from the car, picking up the baby, carrying a toddler—all need to be considered separately. Often a reapportionment of duties among other household members plus financial arrangements for the washing and ironing will solve the major problems, but part-time or full-time housekeeping help may be necessary.

The location and arrangement of the housing, with attention to the amount of climbing and walking required, and the adequacy of labor-saving appliances, are important factors in determining the arrangements and expenditures necessary.

No economy is as great as keeping a mother alive and able to take care of her children. The time and funds necessary for working out small details are savings no community can afford to overlook.

Wage earners whose regular jobs are suited to their physical condition after a heart attack do not generally come to the attention of a welfare department. Those with whom the agency is concerned are the men whose former occupations require physical exertions beyond the capacity of a damaged heart. Vocational rehabilitation is, thus, always a consideration, except for clients in chronic congestive failure, those with complications, and those with extremely severe disease. Referral to the vocational rehabilitation agency should be made when the physician gives his permission and when the client is emotionally ready to accept it. Pushing him against his will is, of course, ineffectual as well as damaging.

When the rehabilitation training or job placement plan

is being made, coöperating social workers must think of the details involved. How will the client get to the place of work? Will he have to stand out on a cold, windy corner waiting for a ride, and, if so, does he have the warm socks, heavy jacket, wool shirt that he needs? Will he have to walk a mile in the scorching sun of summer? Does his wife know how to prepare a low-salt, low-fat, low-calorie lunch of sufficient palatability and nourishment to get him through the day? If not, who can help her?

Will the client have to try to compete for the first time in a world that is strange and anxiety-rousing to him? Have we added exertions and worries at this point by our requirements for budget recomputation, for errands to get receipts for verification of special needs, for adjusting for overpayments? How many blocks does he have to walk to the welfare office, and how long does he have to wait? Do his doctor and the rehabilitation counselor know the realities that must be included in their measurement of the amount of strain the client is under?

Conferences are time consuming, and "teams" sometimes do not produce true team play. Consequently, we tend to avoid them; but rehabilitation of the client with heart disease almost requires that the physician, counselor, and social worker get together, sometimes more than once. Frequently, it is up to the social worker to think of the "little things" that make the difference between whether a plan is workable or not, to ask the questions that help the others to realize the practical aspects, and to cope with the annoying and time-consuming details.

Conferences are often frustrating in another way, by showing that goals for specific clients are not attainable until more community resources have been created, and this usually involves explanation of need to higher authorities and to lay people of influence.

REST

Rest is paramount for the cardiac. It is a deceptively easy-sounding term, but if the springs are broken in the sofa, the mattress lumpy and thin, the house crowded, or the family atmosphere sullen, the client will have a hard time resting. The recommendation for rest may necessitate provision of a separate bed and of more bedding for him, or it may even necessitate the family's moving to a larger house.

In order that the client have emotional rest, the social worker may need to consider services to other members of the family, such as clinic treatment for a crying child's running ear, emotional support or a washing machine for an overburdened wife, a Boy Scout membership for a worrisome predelinquent.

Fundamental in achieving relaxation is emotional security —the complete assurance that shelter and food and minimum essentials will be available, and that thoughtful medical care is quickly accessible. Categorical aid provisions for regular continuing grants as opposed to emergency assistance fill the first security need and, consequently, should be processed as quickly as posible if the client seems to be eligible. When general assistance is the only available source of aid, the client should know that he can count on the check, and will not have to worry each month about whether he can pay the rent.

In considering the extent to which a relative has met any liability the client may have, the amount the relative has expended in emergency medical situations should be considered where policy permits. Heart attacks are frightening not only for the client but for the family, and most persons in an emergency are likely to encumber themselves for items, conducive to relief of anxiety and to the sick person's comfort, which in the cold light of day may prove to have been beyond their means. They call unauthorized physicians if they cannot get hold of the customary doctor, take taxis to hospitals, get drugs from the nearest drugstore, make long-distance calls, make arrangements for luxuries for the patient. Where flexibility in budgeting is possible, this human response to illness must be taken into account.

Security for medical care may or may not be an item the public assistance agency can provide. To the patient, this security is essentially a matter of knowing that he can obtain competent medical care and medication when he needs it. It depends on many factors, such as whether a telephone can be included in the budget, whether the client is entitled to private medical care from public assistance funds, on municipal or county hospital staffing and procedures, on the medical consultant in the agency, the personality of the client's own doctor, and the personality of the client and family.

Medical "shopping" may prove a problem when the client feels that the first doctor he sees is not helpful, or if his anxiety is such that he is compelled to keep trying to find reassurance. In a large county where the worker does not know the medical personnel involved, she can sometimes help in securing the coöperation of an understanding physician through information obtained from the social service department of the municipal or county hospital, or from the agency medical social or medical consultant. In a small community the client usually knows the physicians by reputation and makes his own choice. If not, the worker usually knows the medical personalities well enough so that she can seek out a physician who considers the "total person," and can arrange for the client to see him to get the interpretation and supervision he needs.

DIET

Diet is a difficult matter in heart disease, and may be restricted in salt, fat, total calories, or a combination of all these. The family which has used fried potatoes, fried mush, fried eggs, bread, spaghetti, salt pork, and bologna as the mainstays of their diet will have to face a complete readjustment of eating habits. Unsalted oatmeal probably costs no more than fried mush, but palatability prevents the substitution in most instances. Unsalted bread molds quickly, and the inexperienced average housewife does not know how to wash the salt out of margarine.

The public health nurse can do much in teaching the homemaker the kind of diet that is indicated. Clinic dietitians and home economists with the agriculture department are also resources. The Heart Association has printed material of great value.

Special diets are costly, owing to transportation for the shopping around necessary to create palatable food, and owing to the fact that most low-cost meats are both salty and high in fat content. Fresh fruits and vegetables used in lieu of carbohydrate fillers are also costly.

Workers in the aid to dependent children, aged, and disabled programs, in which most of cardiac clients are found, should equip themselves with knowledge of the practical problems of heart disease diets, and should arrange for experts to talk with the homemaker; if this is not possible, the worker should plan to discuss foods and diet shopping.

WARMTH

Sufficient warmth to avoid chilling is one of the fundamental needs of the cardiac. The down to earth need for enough clothing and bedding and for a sufficient allowance for utilities, strangely enough, may present the worker with her greatest difficulty in helping the recipient, because policy may not permit desirable budgetary adaptations.

However, there are some things the worker can do. First, she should make sure that the recipient is receiving the maximum to which he is entitled under the limitations of the policy. Other members of the household should not be expected to meet the recipient's share of housing and utilities unless they are genuinely able to do so. Frequently the recipient can have a large enough utility item in his budget to meet his particular physical needs if he has been provided with his share.

Second, utilities are often wasted in poorly constructed housing. If this is true, the recipient can be helped to secure housing which better conserves the warmth available. This may mean moving, or in owned homes it may mean repairs and remodeling.

Third, private agency resources may be utilized for clothing, bedding, heaters, if these items cannot be met within the grant. Church groups and similar small organizations usually respond well to requests for such items when need is obviously related to a serious health problem.

Emotional Problems

The emotional concomitants of heart disease range from denial of its existence to unnecessary bedfastness. Conscious and unconscious importance are attached to the heart.

One of the symptoms of heart disease, dyspnea (shortness of breath), has been described under pulmonary emphysema and asthma as the most frightening of all physical states. The heart has been vested with both conscious and unconscious importance. A twinge which would not be noticed if it were in the stomach or the foot is likely to cause panic if it occurs in the left chest, because of our knowledge of life's dependence on the heart. The painfulness of severe angina and of myocardial infarctions is such as to deserve the fear that is felt about another attack.

Some persons react to overwhelming fear by pretending that the condition does not exist. To acknowledge it would be to have to face something they cannot face. Denial is sometimes thought of as courage, as a commendable attitude, but actually it is unhealthy. In order to take advantage of the limited help which can be provided to heart disease patients, and especially in order to live intelligently within cardiac restrictions, the patient needs to accept his disease and his limitations.

The social worker encounters denial most frequently in young men or adolescents who cannot tolerate restriction during a stage of personality development which is normally a time of emancipation, or in emotionally immature adults. Whereas we cannot change personalities, we can avoid reinforcing unhealthy attitudes by not encouraging employment which is contraindicated and by not accepting the client's own statement of his health at face value.

Contrary to the, unfortunately, favorable response to a client who uses denial, a common response to the client with excessive fear is that his fear is shameful, or that the client is trying to get something for nothing by acting more ill than he is. Whereas we do occasionally encounter a malingerer or a hypochondriac, most of our clients are either justifiably afraid, or they are over-reacting because of excessive pain caused by anxiety's physiological response, or they have been misinformed about the implications of their condition. A good physician whom the client trusts is the best remedy.

Cardiac neuroses are usually severe emotional disturbances set down on top of some cardiac disease or sometimes on none at all. The difference between a cardiac neurosis and organic cardiac disease which does not show up via laboratory tests may be slight, and mistakes in diagnosis do occur. Assuming that an accurate diagnosis of cardiac neurosis has been made, the ideal remedy is highly skilled, long-time psychotherapy. If a mental hygiene clinic is available, and will accept the client, he may be helped. Otherwise, an attempt should be made to secure psychiatric consultation. The client is usually a dependent person, and emotional dependency requires great patience and tolerance on the part of the worker. The client's pains may be emotionally induced, but they and his fears are real.

TERMS FREQUENTLY USED IN MEDICAL REPORTS

Acute failure. A condition in which the heart is rapidly deteriorating in its capacity to maintain life. Not necessarily fatal if medical intervention is available and the heart has the capacity to respond or compensate.

Aneurysm. A widening; a sac formed by the dilatation of the walls of an artery or of a vein and filled with blood.

Angina pectoris. A disease marked by paroxysmal chest pain, with suffocation and dizziness, usually caused by lack of blood to the heart muscle, and precipitated by effort or excitement.

Anoxia. Oxygen deficiency.

Aorta. The main artery or arterial trunk from which the entire arterial system proceeds.

Arrhythmia. Any variation from the normal rhythm of the heart beat.

Arterial. Pertaining to the arteries.

Ascites. An accumulation of fluid in the abdomen caused by inadequate function of the circulatory system.

Atherosclerosis. Accumulation of fatty deposits in the arteries

Atrium. An auricle of the heart.

Auricles. The upper chambers of the heart which serve as collecting stations for the blood.

Bundle branch block. A condition in which one ventricle contracts without the other because of obstruction in one of the branches of the bundles of the heart; also known as *heart block*.

Cardiac. Pertaining to the heart.

Cerebral. Pertaining to the cerebrum, the main part of the brain.

Cholesterol. A fatlike, pearly substance, found in all animal fats and oils, in bile, blood, and brain tissue, which accumulates in the arteries, causing atherosclerosis.

Chronic failure. A condition consisting of bouts of acute failure with intervals of finely balanced compensation, or a condition in which chronic symptoms demonstrate that the heart's activity is at low ebb.

Congestive failure. Technically, an overfullness of the blood vessels of an organ or part. The term is used to describe the serious condition in which the heart is not keeping up with the demands upon it.

Coronary. Refers to the vessels which fit over the heart and provide nourishment for its muscle.

Coronary insufficiency. Insufficient provision of blood by the arteries to the tissues of the heart.

Coronary thrombosis. The formation of a clot, in a branch of the coronary arteries which supply blood to the heart muscle, causing obstruction of the artery.

Diastolic. Pertaining to diastole or the resting phase of the heart beat.

Dicumarol. One of the drugs which are anticoagulants or blood thinners.

Digitalis. A cardiac stimulant; a heart tonic for cardiac weakness of any kind.

Dilatation. The condition of being dilated or stretched beyond the normal dimensions.

Dyspnea. Difficult or labored breathing.

Fb. (fingerbreadth). The breadth of a finger.

Fibrillation. Action of the heart muscle in which the various groups of its muscle fibers beat independently and without rhythm.

Heparin. A quick-acting anticoagulant.

Hepatic. Pertaining to the liver.

Hypertension. High blood pressure. *Essential h.* High blood pressure without known cause. *Benign h.* Essential hypertension which exists for years without producing symptoms. *Malignant h.* Essential hypertension with an acute, stormy onset, a rapidly progressive course, and a poor prognosis.

Hypertrophy. Enlargement or overgrowth of an organ or part.

Hypoxia. Deficiency of oxygen.

Ischemia. Deficiency of blood to a part, such as to the heart muscle.

Mitral stenosis. A scarring of the mitral valve.

Mitral valve. The valve between the left auricle and the left ventricle.

Myocardial infarction. Death of a part of the heart muscle.

Myocardium. The heart muscle.

Occlusion. The act of closure or the state of being closed; in coronary disease, the clogging of a vessel by a clot.

Orthopnea. Inability to breathe except in an upright position.

Pericardium. The membranous sac which contains the heart.

Peripheral. Situated at or near the outer part or surface.

Rales. Abnormal sounds in the lungs heard through the stethoscope.

Renal. Pertaining to the kidney.

Retinopathy. Technically, a noninflammatory disease of the retina; refers to one of the complications which occur as an end result of hypertension or of diabetes.

Systolic. Pertaining to the systole or the pushing part of the heart beat.

Tachycardia. A heart pulse rate of above 100 per minute; excessively rapid action of the heart.

Thrombosis. A clot in a blood vessel or in the heart.

Vascular. Pertaining to or full of blood vessels.

Vasoconstriction. The diminution of the caliber of blood vessels

CHAPTER XII

Cerebral Vascular Disease

CEREBRAL (meaning "brain") VASCULAR (pertaining to blood vessels) DISEASE occurs as the consequence of several disorders. The major manifestations are *cerebral vascular accidents* (CVA's or strokes) and *cerebral arteriosclerosis* (a gradual hardening of the arteries of the brain). The discussion here will confine itself to these two conditions.

Cerebral vascular disease is such a widespread condition that almost all social workers have firsthand experience with it either in their caseloads or among their relatives. The disorder causes the greatest number of deaths next to heart disease and cancer, is responsible for an untold amount of crippling, and ranks as the next to greatest cause of first admissions to mental hospitals.

More women than men are said to have cerebral vascular disease. Mental impairments that are caused by cerebral arteriosclerosis occur in later life, most after fifty-five years of age. Strokes can occur at any age, but most persons who have them are more than sixty-five years old.

CVA's or strokes frequently leave both physical and mental *residuals,* or aftereffects. The physical effects are predominantly one-sided paralysis (*hemiplegia*) and impairment of speech (*aphasia*). These present medical and social problems of an entirely different nature than do the mental impairments of cerebral arteriosclerosis, but because the combined effects, bodily and mental, of cerebral vascular disease often exist in the same person they are treated together in this chapter.

A state of flux exists in the understanding and treatment of cerebral vascular disease which causes confusion but which also inspires. Great advances have been recently made in the medical management of patients who have had a CVA. Many hemiplegics, who earlier would have been doomed to vegetative life in bed, can now be restored to at least a modicum of usefulness and independence.

A breakthrough has also come in the treatment of persons with the mental impairments of old age. The disoriented and listless sometimes can now be returned to a state of orientation and greatly improved vigor. As will be discussed later, the physiological effects of cerebral arteriosclerosis and other physical aspects of aging and the psychological and social effects of aging are all so intertwined in their effects upon the functioning of the brain that it is not known what to credit to physical and what to mental causation and remedy. The behavior of the person is truly psychosomatic or unified physical and psychological response. Good medical-social management often brings great and sometimes dramatic improvement.

Thus, social workers of today can approach the problem of clients with cerebral vascular disease with conviction that their efforts will often improve the client's independence, happiness, and well-being. Yet, the problems are still formidable, and require patience, provision for good medical management, adequate resources, and attention to detail. The worker can, however, bring honest optimism to her responsibilities.

General Medical Base for Social Planning

PHYSIOLOGICAL BACKGROUND

In thinking about what happens to an individual physically, it helps to keep in mind a few simple facts about the neurological and circulatory systems. The brain, it will be recalled, is the commander-in-chief of the body; as such, it has first priority on the blood pumped by the heart for the very good reason that it will die unless it receives a constant supply of blood-borne oxygen.

The vessels which supply the brain have branches, and the branches twigs, which create a fine network of tiny vessels. Two large arteries, the *common carotids,* originate directly or indirectly from the aorta and come up along the right and left side of the throat, and subdivide into *external* and *internal carotid arteries*. At the back of the head, the *vertebral* arteries from the spinal column join to form the *basilar* artery, which gives rise to the *posterior cerebrals*. These major arteries and their branches nourish the muscles of the face and throat and the tissues of the brain and skull.

Blood vessels themselves, originally supple, elastic pipes, are subject to injury and stress caused by infections, tension, hormonal imbalance, and obesity, resulting in deposits of fatty substance (*lipids*) forming *atherosclerotic plaques*.

The vessels gradually harden (become *arteriosclerotic*) at a slower or faster pace depending on heredity, diet, exercise, stress, and inflammation from infections. Oddly enough, in spite of the generalized metabolic causes, and although correlations have been shown between damage to the coronary and the cerebral vessels, blood vessels do not deteriorate at a uniform rate throughout the body. One or more blood vessels can be in bad condition, and others remain normal, evidently depending on local trauma or stress. Thus, a person with atherosclerosis of the vessels of the legs may not have vascular deposits in the brain, and vice versa.

One of several things may happen to the blood vessels of the brain as they become hardened, thickened, or otherwise diseased. They may rupture, spilling blood out into surrounding tissue. Hemorrhage of this sort in an older person is nearly always due to high blood pressure. Or the vessels can be blocked by an *embolus* which has traveled up from the heart or elsewhere when the individual has heart disease or some other pertinent condition. Most frequently, however, they become blocked (*occluded*) by the hardened, fatty deposits of atherosclerosis, or a clot forms at the site of a hardened plaque.

CEREBRAL VASCULAR ACCIDENTS

Sudden blockage from an embolus or occlusion, or from a rupture with hemorrhage, can occur in large or small vessels anywhere in the brain, and can occur in different places at different times or at the same time. Obviously, damage to a large vessel—to a main branch—will do much more harm than damage to a twig. Blockage can either be sudden, or take place gradually.

Blockage or rupture have both an immediate local and a surrounding effect. A widespread neurologic shock occurs, the immediately surrounding area becomes inflamed, causing swelling in the brain tissue or *cerebral edema,* and the area fed by the vessel dies.

If the patient survives (which is more likely to occur in occlusion than in hemorrhage) and is kept quiet and receives the medical and nursing attention he needs, the shock gradually wears off and the inflammation or edema of surrounding tissues abates so that they can function with varying degrees of normality again. The immediate tissue which was fed by the blocked or ruptured vessel, of course, cannot revive; brain tissue once destroyed cannot regenerate.

However, the functions carried on by that bit of tissue may be partly taken over by some other part of the brain. Compensatory circulation may sometimes be established through new channels quickly enough to keep partly damaged tissue from complete destruction. Some form of reorganization in the functioning of the total brain seems to occur, which evidently is still not completely understood.

The brain's responsibility is to receive, sort out, and direct messages to muscles, thought, sensation, and speech through geographical functional compartmentalization. Thus the death of, or temporary damage to, certain tissues may cause any of various kinds of outward or neurologic symptoms. The most frequent are one-sided paralysis (*hemiplegia*), language inability (*aphasia*), seizures (*epilepsy*), difficulty in swallowing, complete or partial loss of vision (the most common partial form being one called *hemianopsia*), incontinence, dizziness (*vertigo*), and mental impairment characterized by intellectual deterioration and emotional instability.

Onset and Initial Care

Although it is possible for a stroke to occur in stages, a major stroke usually happens suddenly with a partial or complete loss of consciousness. A medical emergency exists when coma is present. The person should be under constant professional supervision either in a hospital or by arrangement for medical care and round-the-clock nursing at home. His life is in jeopardy, and he needs various medical procedures and careful nursing care. In selected cases in medical centers which have the facilities, surgical procedures may sometimes be employed.

The physician will try to determine the cause of the stroke, as well as take emergency lifesaving measures, because the prognosis and later treatment depend on a knowledge of what brought it on. About 25 per cent of CVA's are said to be caused by hemorrhages due to high blood pressure in diseased arteries; the outlook in these cases is grave. If the patient who has had a hemorrhage does survive, his exercises and ambulation cannot be started as early as if he had had an occlusion. He will need a longer period of rest and close medical supervision.

If a client who has had a stroke cannot be hospitalized, the worker should be aware that one of the essentials in his care at home is absolute quiet for the first week or two, which may require emergency social arrangements. Another essential is that he be turned frequently to avoid pneumonia and bedsores.

Because catheterization and proper positioning in bed are involved, and because appropriate exercises will have to be started soon, some kind of nursing is necessary, ideally by a nurse who understands the simple but important modern rehabilitation procedures. The pillows, pulleys, sandbags, and other equipment needed will, like provision for personal services, frequently mean immediate budget adjustments.

Anxiety-producing situations should be avoided for the first six months. The social worker's role in accomplishing this goal may be substantial.

Outlook for Recovery

Whether the person survives, how soon he returns to consciousness, and what extent and kind and permanence of neurologic effects he will have, all depend on the cause of the stroke and where it took place in the brain, the existence of other complications, and the care he receives. The longer he stays unconscious, the less chance he has to survive. The extent of the immediate paralysis does not indicate the extent of future disability. Paralysis, blindness, difficulty in swallowing, inability to recognize words or to speak, may all clear up if they were caused by shock and transient edema and not by actual tissue destruction.

Experts can make reliable predictions within the first few days in some cases, but time is usually required before the doctor can determine the extent and kind of permanent disability. Conservative estimates are that six months should elapse before a decision is made regarding the extent of permanent damage. Even two or three years later, functional improvement in the use of paralyzed limbs can occur if the person has the mentality, motivation, and opportunity for the right kind of instruction.

The likelihood of another stroke exists, of course, if the underlying cause is not one that can be brought under control. In a few isolated cases, where the stroke was caused by an injury, the future may be free from vascular hazard; where the stroke was caused by inadequately treated high blood pressure, which can be controlled by diet, medication, and rest, there are grounds for hope that another stroke can be avoided for an indefinite period.

As has been discussed, most strokes are, however, caused by plugs or occlusion from atherosclerosis (with or without high blood pressure) and, unfortunately, there are no known sure means at this time of preventing them. Various drugs are used, but according to the literature none are markedly effective with the exception of the *anticoagulants* (blood thinners), such as *heparin* and *dicumarol,* which can be administered only when the patient has access to close medical and laboratory supervision.

Consequently, the patient's fear that he will have another stroke may be well founded. This is less true in older persons than in younger ones; in the younger, not the inevitable consequences of aging but some pathological cause for the speeding up of the "aging" process in the arteries is thought to be to blame. The widely expressed fear that the third stroke will be fatal is an old wives' tale. The size and location of the artery involved, not the number of times a stroke has occurred, determine the outcome. Many persons have a long series of small strokes as will be discussed later.

Hemiplegia

A major stroke frequently produces an immediate paralysis of the side of the body opposite to the brain lesion. Because half the body is involved, it is called *hemiplegia*. When paralysis is less than complete and weakness rather than complete loss of motion occurs, it is technically called *hemiparesis*. The extremities are limp or *flaccid* the first day or so, and then become tight or *spastic*. The face and tongue may be involved, with the mouth and, sometimes, the eyelid drawn down. The shoulder characteristically stiffens and frequently dislocates downward, the elbow and wrist are bent, and the fingers are drawn into the palm. The hip may be stiffened and the leg paralyzed; with a tendency for the foot or the toes to drop down unless a footboard is put across the bed and the feet propped against it to prevent this *drop-foot* deformity.

To prevent deformities and *disuse atrophy* (wasting from lack of exercise), authorities now advocate that within twenty-four hours after a stroke certain preventive rehabilitative measures should be taken—such as putting pillows or sandbags against the outside of the involved leg to keep it from turning outward, and massaging the arm and putting a pillow under the armpit to keep the shoulder in place.

Because our shoulders are more important than we realize in self-care, and because the affected shoulder tends to stiffen quickly, the patient is often taught to raise the paralyzed arm above his head with the help of his good arm. Sometimes a rubber ball is put in the paralyzed hand and the person is encouraged to try to squeeze it, so as to exercise his fingers and keep from digging his nails deeper and deeper into his palm.

Getting up in a chair at the earliest possible time, which is one of the rehabilitation goals, has physical and mental advantages. Man was intended to maintain a vertical position; the body chemistry actually goes awry if the horizontal plane is assumed for a prolonged period, a fact incorporated in the current emphasis on early postoperative ambulation. The paralyzed person is in double jeopardy from lying flat because his circulation is poor. Bedsores (*decubitus ulcers*) add needless, burdensome complications.

Once the person is up in a chair, he is encouraged to pull himself up to a standing position, and then to take steps with the help of appliances and parallel bars, and even to walk up and down stairs.

The incontinence of many hemiplegic patients is considered by some authorities to be due to brain damage, and by others to the horizontal position plus apathy and despair or to loss of self-respect through loss of independence.

No one can gainsay the good mental and physical results of keeping patients stimulated, having them move about, doing as much as they possibly can for themselves, learning new ways of overcoming dependence, and remaining in an optimistic frame of mind. Overcoming incontinence, greatly facilitated by the ability to get to the commode, results in

a lesser burden on the family, increases positive relationships and promotes self-respect in the patient.

Mental impairments following strokes vary in extent of
severity and permanence, just as do the outward physical
manifestation of brain damage. The tendency to cry on
slight provocation (excessive *emotional lability*) is such
a common feature that it is sometimes regarded as part of
the clinical picture following a CVA; it is one of the most
humiliating and vocationally handicapping impairments.
Nervousness, instability, and slight to severe mental deterioration are also often present.

Mental and physical rehabilitation are interdependent.
Alleviation of physical frustrations, hopefulness, and lessened physical dependence relieve the distressed mental state
and increase self-control. However, extensive brain lesions,
especially those in certain areas, actually prevent learning,
no matter how well motivated the recipient may be or how
intelligent he was before the accident.

Optimistic estimates are made that 90 per cent of
hemiplegics could learn to walk if rehabilitation measures
were begun immediately and continued under skilled supervision. Physicians vary in their estimates of the numbers
who can attain self-care skills.

The prognosis is influenced primarily by the size and location of the destroyed brain tissue, by how quickly rehabilitation measures are started, by the person's motivation and
circumstances, and by the amount and duration of mental
impairment.

From a practical standpoint, the prognosis depends in
part on whether the recipient gets the right kind of medical
and nursing home care. Physical restoration measures must
be guided by a physician. The underlying condition or the
cause of the stroke should be treated in part to minimize
the chances of recurrence. The extent of exercise which can

be tolerated has to be correlated with the general physical condition; drugs must be regulated and concurrent problems treated.

The many assistive devices and home aids and the use of exercises are relatively new, and require highly specialized knowledge. Physicians who are expert in physical restoration are called physiatrists. Many teaching centers now have departments of physical medicine. Physicians frequently use the technical help of a rehabilitation-oriented nurse or physical or occupational therapist in devising and carrying out restoration programs.

The knowledge, attitudes, and available time of the nursing home operator or, if the person is in his own home, of the major caretaker, also vitally affect physical restoration. Infinite patience and tact are required in dealing with the often fearful, slow-moving, deeply discouraged patient. Both conviction and special knowledge are essential; again the rehabilitation-oriented nurse or the therapist is a helpful ally.

Prognosis is equally determined by whether the recipient has the means and the environment to secure the things that are often taken for granted: quiet, peace of mind, cleanliness, stout shoes and other essential clothing, bedding, security, the right kind of diet, hope for the future, a wheel chair, transportation to the clinic.

Aphasia

Loss of language (*aphasia*) is unfortunately one of the common results of cerebral vascular accidents, and is one of the least understood and most inadequately managed medical problems. Aphasia is caused by a lesion on the "dominant" (usually left) side, and is often accompanied by right-sided hemiplegia. There are, of course, other causes of loss of speech: congenital deafness with mutism or removal of the voice box (*laryngectomy*) in the treatment of cancer.

Of all sensory losses, inability to communicate is said to be the most defeating and depressing. Because it is such a severe disability, from both emotional and realistic viewpoints, we may be grateful that in many cases aphasia is only partial, and that in many cases it clears up spontaneously within several months.

Aphasia is referred to as *global* if it is total, as *expressive* if it refers to speaking and writing only, and *receptive* if it refers to understanding and reading only. There are technical terms for certain aspects of aphasia, such as *agraphia* for inability to write and *alexia* for inability to read.

A stroke can also cause paralysis of the muscles involved in speech (*dysarthria*). It is not quite so handicapping as aphasia, because if the motor control centers of the brain which affect the speech muscles rather than the language control centers have been damaged or destroyed, the person can at least write out or point to what he wants. He obviously is less handicapped than the person whose brain refuses to associate words with objects at all.

A properly trained speech therapist or an expert physician can evaluate whether the problem is aphasia or dysarthria. It is important that this differentiation be made, because remedial training differs for the two problems. A further diagnostic matter of the utmost importance is differentiating aphasic patients from psychotic or demented ones. If a person has receptive aphasia—that is, if he cannot understand what is being said to him and cannot translate what his environment is telling him about where he is or who he is—great danger exists that he will be thought to be suffering from dementia.

The person who can understand, but who cannot express

himself because words elude him, may be so upset and frustrated and frightened by his plight that he may behave as though he were mentally impaired. This is particularly true unless the aphasia is carefully explained to him, so that he knows what has happened and can see that treatment is being started to help him.

The person who has had a stroke which leaves him silent and seemingly uncomprehending must not be written off as a vegetable and placed in an institution to die. If he has wealth and access to experts, the danger is less than in the case of the public assistance recipient receiving scanty medical care, who may have no one but the social worker to raise questions and stimulate arrangements for such expert evaluation and treatment as is available.

In aphasia which is not the result of shock or edema, but rather is caused by destruction of tissue—in other words, which does not clear up naturally—the prognosis for learning a complete vocabulary is poor. The language centers in the dominant cerebral hemisphere (that which controls our "handedness") has been destroyed, and the only remaining function is that which is on the minor side. The minor side is weak and subject to almost immediate fatigue at first. The gradual strengthening of the minor side is the physiological goal of training efforts.

In spite of poor prognosis for complete return of language through relearning, a vocabulary sufficient for at least adequate limited communication is possible in many cases. Normal language—not a language substitute—is taught, so that the patient can hope eventually to communicate with others than his caretakers.

Emphasis is placed on teaching specific words such as "bread" rather than collective or general words such as "food." The teaching begins with words most necessary and meaningful to the patient, such as "water," "toilet," "bed." Nouns are taught first, as they are thought to be the easiest to learn.

The training requires many months, and sometimes years, of patient, kindly effort, because relearning takes place by repetition in an emotionally advantageous climate. The family and volunteers can help, with the advice and supervision of a speech therapist. The aphasic individual who has right-sided hemiplegia may be taught to write with his left hand. Something about writing words helps the brain register them. The patient is encouraged to listen to radio and to watch television, and to look at picture magazines and newspapers, even though he cannot understand the words.

There are many peculiarities about aphasia: a patient may be able to say certain words at certain times but not at others, or he may be able to swear or to sing but not to talk. The reorganization of brain functioning after damage is not completely understood. Restoration of language is extraordinarily complex, because language requires recognition, memory, recall, formulation, and motor accomplishments, all of which involve different parts of the brain.

Experience has, however, demonstrated the importance of brief but frequent speech therapy sessions, avoidance of fatigue, an optimistic atmosphere, opportunity for the person to express himself no matter how imperfectly or how slowly, and patience on the part of family, therapist, social worker, and physician. The mental capacity of the patient has the same bearing upon relearning as upon original learning.

Small Strokes or Multiple Cerebral Thromboses

A series of small strokes, not infrequently beginning in middle age, is a common result of cerebral arteriosclerosis. Small blood vessels break or occlude in different parts of the brain, causing a variety of transient physical symptoms and usually resulting in personality changes or mental deterioration.

These small strokes (sometimes called pinpoint strokes) may not be identified as such by either the patient or the physician. They do not necessarily create unconsciousness or any type of paralysis but rather may be manifested by sudden giddiness, weakness, nausea, diarrhea, or "jolts," followed by continued burning sensations in the abdomen, loss of weight, or other, sometimes bizarre, feelings of misery. The episode usually ends after a few hours, often leaving no tangible, measurable effect which a doctor can detect on examination, but frequently leaving the person feeling depressed and miserable.

When small strokes are identified, the patient may be apprehensive about further, more serious ones. Whereas the apprehension is justified, many persons do go for years without more; then too, the subsequent ones, like the first, may be in small vessels in relatively unimportant locations in the brain so far as physical functions are concerned. Thus the social worker can honestly reinforce the physician's optimistic interpretation to the recipient while knowing that the prognosis is generally poor.

The not infrequent result of small strokes is permanent mental impairment. Noticeable personality change, untidiness, apathy, or general deterioration with lack of capacity for work and concentration, loss of memory, insomnia, periods of confusion, restlessness, or loss of judgment, may follow a small stroke or series of strokes. Dr. Walter Alvarez tells of examining an important executive referred to him for consultation by another doctor, who later telephoned and asked, "What did you find?" Dr. Alvarez quotes himself as saying "Gravy on his vest." *

---

* Walter Alvarez, "Cerebral Arteriosclerosis," *Geriatrics* I (May–June, 1946), 203.

Dr. Alvarez further points out that one of the kindest things the doctor can do for the patient is to treat the family. If the recipient does not have a physician who spontaneously assumes the responsibility of interpreting to the patient's family what has happened so that they can understand unexplained, unwelcome behavior as illness rather than as "orneriness," the social worker may need to ask the physician for this service.

Treatment varies according to the physician's preference. None is known at this time which will repair the damage to the brain. If the arteriosclerosis is complicated by other diseases such as diabetes or hypertension, as often happens, the physician will attempt to bring these into control. He may prescribe anticoagulant medicine to thin the blood and try to prevent further thromboses. Excesses of all kinds are advised against, including those of worry and physical activity. Most physicians are strict about diet and smoking, but others feel that the patient may indulge to help him stay as happy as he can, in view of the limited amount medical science can do at this time to prevent further deterioration or to postpone death.

CEREBRAL ARTERIOSCLEROSIS

Cerebral arteriosclerosis (hardening of the arteries of the brain) causes varying degrees of mental impairment designated by laymen as senility but technically classified as chronic brain syndrome associated with cerebral arteriosclerosis, or as chronic brain syndrome associated with senile brain disease. There are differences in these two classifications; further, cerebral arteriosclerosis is not synonymous with senility. However, the terms are used so loosely and interchangeably, and the scientific differences are so difficult to distinguish at this stage of knowledge, that the loose interpretation of cerebral arteriosclerosis will be used in this discussion.

Still other terms to be found on medical reports for the same entity are *chronic brain syndrome, encephalomalacia, generalized arteriosclerosis* (usually abbreviated as G.A.S.), *senile psychosis, senile brain disease, senile dementia,* and *cortical atrophy.*

Cerebral arteriosclerosis is actually a condition in which the small arteries of the brain narrow in caliber and bore. They more or less harden and become plugged, so that the blood can no longer get through well to bathe the tissues with needed oxygen and other nutrients. This general impairment of the circulation of the brain results in a symptom complex of irritability, forgetfulness, emotional instability, tremor, and muscular weakness.

Senile brain disease, which arises from all the physiological and psychical effects of aging, creates symptoms ranging from childishness to complete vegetation. It is usually characterized by lack of clarity in orientation, impairment in judgment and reasoning, and sometimes by impulsive or violent behavior with paranoid trends.

Diffuse, increasing brain damage from widespread cerebral arteriosclerosis also has much in common with the mental impairment from one or a series of strokes or vascular thromboses. We would expect to find a major difference in behavior when one or more small, circumscribed, isolated sections of tissue die, compared with behavior when a wide area is slowly dying; but because the brain acts in a coördinated manner, damage to one part can interfere with the functioning of the rest, simulating a diffuse impairment.

Until recently, the characteristic behavior of cerebral arteriosclerosis and/or senile brain disease was considered due entirely to physical cause. These diseases were considered progressive and not amenable to correction. However, recent experiments which have compared behavior in life with the appearance of brains at autopsy show that the assumed correlation does not exist. Some persons whose behavior has been senile show little brain pathology; conversely, some with extensive damage to the arteries did not behave in a markedly senile manner.

Further, experience has shown that the behavior of many "senile" persons is greatly affected by both physical and social problems, including diet. Nutrition is believed to be an important factor. Particular reference is made to vitamin intake and the effects of anemia.

If a person is anemic, the poor quality of the blood which does get through the impaired vessels to the brain tissues diminishes the supply of oxygen, thus aggravating the physiological cause of symptoms. The same is true if heart disease impairs the blood supply to the brain, or if the blood lacks enough sugar, or if it clots too readily.

Recent experience of social agencies and mental hospitals also demonstrates that senile behavior is influenced by the social situation of the person. The comments of a nurse are especially sensitive in describing an old person's situation:

The normal young person bulwarked by good health, surrounded by loved ones, happy in his busy daily routine, free in his ability to function independently, secure as an integrated whole, can, "without falling apart," adjust and cope with stress, anxiety, and unexpected emergencies. In contrast, let's view the pathetic oldster with failing powers, loss of vision, poor hearing, weak gait, and faulty memory, whose loved ones are deceased, whose days are spent doing little that is rewarding or purposeful, possibly surrounded by disinterested strangers. To this person stress in a form as simple as an imagined grievance can build up into a tremendous crisis resulting in behavior described as unmanageable, argumentative, uncoöperative, belligerent, irascible, quarrelsome, destructive, and psychotic.[2]

Aging itself carries emotional burdens, especially in our culture which glorifies vigor and youth. The older person is often socially isolated, feels neglected—and with good cause—is insecure, anxious, and depressed. He needs to be able to lean emotionally on someone more and more as his own physical independence weakens. The person he formerly leaned on may have died, or may have a home and interests of his own. The financial, ego, and companionship satisfactions which he formerly secured from work may also have disappeared.

Therefore cerebral arteriosclerosis or the physical concomitant of aging is coincidentally accompanied by severe social and emotional problems. A vicious circle occurs when depression reduces food intake and thus adds to the danger of anemia which, in turn, increases the severity of the oxygen deprivation to the cortex. The emotions literally produce a physiological effect on behavior.

The social and emotional factors in the total response of the individual who has cerebral arteriosclerosis probably offer greater opportunity for modification than do the physical results of the disease, but it is difficult to separate what is physiological from what is psychological response. Pleasant surroundings, good mental hygiene, adequate diet, useful activity, moderate exercise, pursuit of interests, reassurance, and someone who cares—all are important aspects of treatment. The special importance of continued activity and a feeling of usefulness has been emphasized by many authorities.

---

* Blanche D. Gubersky, "Geriatric Nursing," *in* E. V. Cowdry, ed., *The Care of the Geriatric Patient* (St. Louis: C. V. Mosby Co., 1958), p. 217.

A physician who takes an interest in the aged person and who has the temperament for geriatrics can be particularly helpful, if he is not deprived of necessary pharmaceutical tools by financial restrictions. Vitamins, hormonal treatment, attention to bodily miseries that cause mental and physical stress, prescription of diet and activities, attention to serious concomitant conditions such as diabetes and heart disease, and medication directed at the cerebral arteriosclerosis—all constitute the various measures used in medical treatment.

Remarkable improvement in the behavior of senile persons has been achieved by social measures, particularly in the matter of diet. For example, in the "Meals on Wheels" programs, one hot meal a day is taken by volunteers to the homes of aged persons to make sure they are tempted to eat nourishing food and thereby to be less likely to deteriorate and to require mental hospital care.

Emotional upset is known to increase disorganized behavior; conversely, security and content decrease it. Family boarding-home care has become an important means of relieving the stress of loneliness and unmet needs. The success of day-care centers for the aged, Golden Age clubs, and social and recreational programs in board-and-care homes and nursing homes is testimony to the widespread recognition of the palliative effects on senility of relief from emotional stress.

Exercise coupled with usefulness, as in housework or self-care activities, is also known to delay the progress of senility. It is not clearly understood whether the action is physiological, reducing the progress of cerebral arteriosclerosis, or psychological, reducing the total reaction of the brain to hopelessness and unhappiness.

Just as age and degree of cerebral arteriosclerosis do

not correlate, neither does life prognosis correlate with extent of mental impairment.

Persons with cerebral arteriosclerosis frequently have concomitant coronary artery disease or hypertension, and may die from heart disease, diabetes, or from an infection. However, if the patient receives good care and modern medical treatment, and if he is not unhappy, he may live with reasonable comfort for an indefinite period.

Implications for Public Assistance

The recent dramatic advances in the treatment of hemiplegia, the beginnings which are being made in prevention of strokes and in the treatment of aphasia, our widening knowledge of physical and social factors in geriatric rehabilitation, and community anxiety over the increasing number of aged persons and the cost of their care—all have combined rapidly to change the social implications of cerebral vascular disease.

Social workers of this era must, like Janus, look forward and backward at the same time, stimulating more intelligent care of recipients who have been neglected, and at the same time attempting to initiate good care for those who newly manifest symptoms of cerebral vascular disease.

Many county hospitals and nursing homes still have many patients to whom modern therapeutics have not been applied. The needlessly vegetative, incontinent, deformed existence of these individuals is duplicated in the homes of those families who are caring for aged relatives without the medical care, guidance, and social services which could lighten family burdens and bring new hope to the disabled persons.

In the past, social work with the aged dealt largely with guardianship provisions, commission hearings, use of nursing-home beds, county hospital admissions and readmissions, excess personal property accumulation from failure to utilize the assistance grant to meet personal needs, and provisions for burials. Today, efforts to secure active medical care, good diet, dental care, resources for prevention and alleviation of disability, and the happiness and usefulness of the individual are replacing the old traditional social services for persons who have cerebral arteriosclerosis.

Part of the problem cannot be met by individual caseworkers on an individual basis; community organization is required. However, there is much that is directly within the province of the caseworker, and she should make sure that time-consuming and often prosaic but important details are given attention.

COMMUNITY ORGANIZATION

Clients who are lying bedfast, incontinent, and sometimes aphasic, or sit vacuously in their chairs in nursing homes or county hospitals or in their own homes, need individual evaluation. Some are beyond help because of extensive mental impairment, but many are not. Careful social review of the case record of each person should include perusal of the medical report. The worker should ascertain whether the physician seems to have made a comprehensive evaluation and has prescribed treatment which is being carried out or whether only a superficial eligibility examination was made. The social worker should also note whether the record indicates that a doctor regularly visits the patient.

When the annual reinvestigation is made, if not before, an attempt should be made to find out as much as possible, from the recipient and the persons who have direct responsibility for taking care of him, about the extent of his physical activity, his interests, habits, personality, speech, incontinence, responses, and alertness. Physical attributes, such as loss of weight, lack of appetite, constipation, bedsores, signs of excessive aging, inadequacy of vision and hearing, are also important to consider in getting a true picture of the patient.

If the patient does not get out of bed, is it because of deformity of the limbs or weakness, or lack of sturdy shoes, or clothes, or lack of time on someone's part to get him up? Does he and does his bed look clean? What does his attitude seem to be toward the attendant or nurse? Does he have visitors?

When only a few clients in the caseload seem to be vegetating, individual measures can be taken to secure an adequate medical appraisal of each, to stimulate a plan for rehabilitation for those who can be helped, and to implement the social measures necessary. If, however, there are a large number, the resources of the county hospital, county health department, voluntary agencies, welfare department, medical society, nursing home association, and other interested community groups need to be pulled together for an attack on the problem of the sick aged as a group.

MEDICAL AND DENTAL CARE

Good medical treatment, frequently including physical restoration services, must be secured for the recipient if he is to have the opportunity for maximum physical improvement. In the many cases where the goal is limited, even a small achievement in improved self-care is meaningful to the recipient and his family.

If the recipient has been crippled by a stroke, the ability to get off the bed onto a chair, or to move about, even with the aid of a walker or wheel chair, to go outdoors, to take care of his own toilet needs, to feed or dress himself, may make the difference between apathy or despair and a feeling of self-worth, between having to stay in an institution or being able to live at home, between functioning and existing as a rejected burden or as a participating member of the family.

Of first importance is medical treatment of underlying conditions, such as high blood pressure, arteriosclerosis, diabetes, heart disease, anemia, and malnutrition. The high cost of drugs, vitamins, and tranquilizers is a serious obstacle to rehabilitation of the aged. The cost to the taxpayer is not wasted, however, if these shorten institutional stays, keep clients on their feet and able to take care of their own needs, and avoid hospital admissions. When the physician recommends body-building drugs, the recipient should be encouraged to secure them and every available resource utilized to assist him.

Special diet is frequently prescribed in the treatment of the common complicating and underlying conditions. The low-calorie, low-fat, low-sodium, and diabetic diets are unpalatable and difficult, as has been discussed earlier. Usually some compromise in the diet must be made if the aged person's lifelong preferences are not to be completely ignored. Near starvation or complete disregard of diet may occur in some congregate living quarters unless the social workers and physicians pay special attention to the food provided to recipients. Recipients living at home and dependent on others for cooking may also have a serious problem unless the worker explores the matter of food habits and preparation, guides the caretaker to any technical help needed, and gives attention to remedying the small practical difficulties that stand in the way of an adequate diet.

Dental care may be the key to an improved physical condition. If teeth are painful or absent, inability to chew may cause a distorted selection of foods, thus defeating adequate nutrition. Unfortunately, securing good dental care, especially for the aged or handicapped, is one of the most stubborn of social problems.

The first essential is to locate dentists who provide quality service for low-income patients. Dental societies, the dental health consultant of the state department of public health, or a socially minded leading dentist in the community can be helpful in providing information.

A dentist's evaluation of the client's needs necessarily precedes any plans for treatment. Transportation to the dentist's office may create a time-consuming problem for the social worker if the client is enfeebled or disabled, and a relative, neighbor, or volunteer must be found to take the client there. A full mouth extraction may prove advisable from a dental standpoint, but be an unsuitable plan unless dentures can be secured.

The dental schools in communities which have them, medical care funds available for dental needs in some states, the client's savings from personal needs provisions of the grant, and aid from relatives are the most usual sources for provision of dentures or extractions. When a direct relationship can be demonstrated between need for dentures and a physical problem, such as stomach ulcers or severe malnutrition, the county or municipal hospital, or a service club may be additional sources of aid.

Unmet dental needs of a large group of clients or recurring problems in meeting dental needs should be brought to the attention of the dental society, the council of social agencies, or other appropriate action groups. Because senior citizen groups often wield substantial influence in local governmental affairs, their leaders may also be helpful in stimulating provision for unmet needs.

CLOTHING

The psychological value of suitable individual clothing for persons in institutions cannot be overestimated for restoring a feeling of self-respect which in itself is the beginning of motivation. A person wearing a nightgown feels like an invalid—someone who has to be cared for. Faded institutional robes and ill-fitting slippers create a feeling of anonymity, bleakness, and lost hope. A person who is dressed in day clothes even though he is lying on a bed, has a sense of identity and a feeling that he is expected to improve.

The need for sturdy shoes is obvious in view of the hemiplegic's problems in relearning to walk. Shoes which give good support and soles which do not tend to turn or slip help prevent falls.

Lack of suitable clothing sometimes creates unwillingness to take advantage of opportunities to attend social and religious gatherings. Relatives or volunteers who will shop for the recipient can often overcome such problems as those caused by inability to wear a corset, by a gain in weight due to immobility, by inability to fasten clothing which fastens in the back.

DEVICES AND EQUIPMENT

The right-sided hemiplegic with substantial arm and hand involvement will have a serious problem in feeding and dressing himself, shaving, combing his hair, opening doors, writing, dialing a telephone, and similar activities on which independence depends.

The most important areas of independence are in eating and in toilet functions.

Assistive devices and specially designed clothing may materially aid the patient in learning to care for himself. They can often be homemade by ingenious relatives or friends or volunteers. *Self-Help Devices for Rehabilitation** tells how to make many of these. Substantial expenditures for special equipment and extra clothing may be necessary in some cases. Fortunately, lay charitable groups often respond well to such needs.

Devices and equipment must be wanted, understood, and trusted in order to be used profitably; they must be tailored to each individual's peculiar muscle weaknesses, living arrangements, and likes and dislikes; often they must be fitted and their use taught in the home. Advanced age and the normal regression of illness intensify problems of using strange new devices or equipment, which are often awkward and require long practice. Persons who are "set in their ways" may seem ungrateful and uncoöperative by offering resistance born of fear, distrust, or dissatisfaction. Much patience is required by all who are participating in the recipient's rehabilitation.

In order to avoid wasteful expenditures, equipment should be tried out before it is purchased, and the recipient should be instructed in its use by either the sales company or a therapist. The often necessary shortening, lengthening, padding, or tightening adjustments should be guaranteed by the sales company. The physician who guides the treatment plan should not only prescribe any equipment but should check it for fit and adequacy. Some experience and/or special training is required before a physician can prescribe this equipment.

Laundry of bed linen of incontinent patients at home is an obviously excessive burden. Providing for it satisfactorily through the budget, after discussion with the caretaker, may go far to delay the day when the recipient must be institutionalized. In many instances, incontinence can be over-

---

* Muriel E. Zimmerman, *Self-Help Devices for Rehabilitation* (Dubuque, Iowa: William C. Brown Co., 1958).

come by rehabilitation measures. The worker should seek help for the family from the physician and public health nurse, rather than indefinitely authorize a special laundry item in the budget.

OTHER NEEDS

Transportation to and from the clinic, doctor's and bracemaker's offices and physical therapy center, may be a substantial special need in cases of hemiplegia, as in other crippling defects. Weekly transportation to a laboratory for blood checkup is necessary when blood thinning medications are being used.

Speech therapy for aphasia can also create a real transportation problem. It is to be remembered that, owing to rapid brain fatigue, the aphasic's therapy has to be provided in short, frequent sessions.

Prevention of falls, with the resultant danger of fractured limbs and further weakening through prolonged bed rest, also requires attention to special needs. Important items for consideration include: a commode beside the bed for use at night, safety rails in the bathroom, light bulbs large enough to facilitate good vision when the person gets up at night, a night light, supportive bedroom slippers, and convenient household arrangements. A homemaker may need to have kitchen shelves lowered, to avoid the danger of falling backward while reaching up and to reduce the temptation to climb. Little things, such as the handiness of the toilet-tissue rack to the toilet, the placement of the mailbox on the porch, are important in helping the aged crippled person avoid falls.

The hemiplegic or senile patient at home should live on the first floor if at all possible, and his sleeping quarters should be near the bathroom. Household rearrangement often merits attention for achieving the greatest degree of convenience for the caretaker and happiness of the recipient.

A comfortable chair and a comfortable mattress are vital to the well-being of people who must spend days, months, or even years sitting or lying down.

Personal services for shampoos, dressing, getting up into a chair or out into the sunshine are frequently needed by the recipient who has any substantial manifestation of cerebral vascular disease. Such services are sometimes lovingly given by a close relative or neighbor, but in many instances, they are not provided at all or are grudgingly given if not paid for. One of the main obstacles to rehabilitation in county institutions and nursing homes is lack of personnel to get people out of bed.

Television and radio are especially important to the homebound person. Through them he can participate in religious services, escape from fear and loneliness, and enjoy recreation. When tubes burn out, as they frequently do when in use, it is important to the recipient to replace them. A daily newspaper with favorite features, such as crossword puzzles, also helps keep the person stimulated and interested in events outside himself, and thus helps to prevent stagnation and deterioration.

LIVING ARRANGEMENTS

The older person with a substantial degree of cerebral vascular disease needs some form of protective care. Some of his personal problems may result from either the fact that he lives alone and needs supervision, or that he lives with relatives to whom he is a burden, or that he lives in an institutional setting which is unsatisfactory to him.

He may be a "difficult" person, confused and stubborn, hostile and excitable, unwilling to take a bath or change clothes, spilling his food, demanding of attention, or excessively dependent. It should be remembered that the behavior of a senile person can often be improved through social measures. Among the foremost of these is the meeting of dependency needs. If the recipient can feel wanted and appreciated and to some extent useful, his behavior may improve to such an extent that planning becomes easier, because more doors are opened to him.

The person who lives alone may have become gradually and almost imperceptibly less capable, making gradual adaptations and living within greater and greater restrictions. Independence and dread of institutional care are common reasons for reluctance to ask for help or to accept suggestions of change.

The right of self-determination extends to all recipients. It is difficult to decide when protection must take precedence over the client's own preferences. Usually the client is aware of his need for protection, is afraid of helplessness or an accident, is lonely and frequently desperate, but he does not have the initiative, capacity for clear thinking, or strength to make a move.

He is torn between his need for help and his desire for independence. A worker who is able to keep in sufficiently close touch with the recipient, so that she can sense when the appropriate time has come for a discussion of institutional care, and who can accept and understand the recipient's ambivalent feelings, backing away from the subject if necessary but returning to it again, is in the best position to help the person take what may be a long-dreaded step.

The importance of little things to the recipient is difficult to appreciate for those who have wide horizons. A compassionate and understanding attempt to respect what is important to the recipient, to give emotional support, and to help the client with the time-consuming minutiae of a change in living plan—all are essential if the recipient's strengths are to be retained for the trials of adjusting to a new setting. The recipient should take some of his own possessions with him, including his favorite chair if at all possible.

Families vary too widely in their attitudes toward aged relatives to make generalizations possible, but ambivalence seems to be the predominant feeling. Rejection of the aged person and the burden he places on the younger, more vigorous members seems almost universal, with a greater or lesser degree of guilt and insight accompanying the feelings of rejection.

Cultural values—strong family feeling, greater respect for the aged—seem to lessen the problem among certain groups, especially the Oriental, Spanish-speaking, and Indian.

Urban families in crowded quarters, those with health problems, or those with unhappy relationships because of other difficulties are least able to adapt to the care of the disabled aged.

Conjugal conflict frequently results if the aged relative of a husband creates a housekeeping and attendant care burden for his wife. The husband is frequently caught in a vise between his filial affection and respect and his wife's hostility, or is troubled by feelings of guilt about the burden his parent creates for his wife. The recipient is unhappy if rejected, and usually prefers to live elsewhere. "Family-centered casework," which is our goal in all cases, means that the needs of each member of the family should be explored and understood as well as possible.

Listening is healing. Persons can often accept difficult situations if they have been given a chance to blow off steam. Hasty action on the basis of violent feeling is to be avoided because the individuals may feel better after they have been interviewed. If, however, rejection, unhappiness, and conflict continue, the recipient should be helped to move.

RELATIONS WITH OTHER HELPING PERSONS

The public health nurse, physician, and clergyman are usually persons vital to the recipient's well-being. The physician often needs the information the social worker has in order fully to understand the client's situation. He can be most helpful with medical-social problems if he has been kept informed and his services are geared with the worker's.

The nurse can advise the family caring for a hemiplegic or senile member about many practical household arrangements and the physical care and mental hygiene of the patient. She may also give emotional support.

The clergyman may not only give the recipient a great deal of comfort and support but serve as a channel to volunteer services for meeting the recipient's social and recreational needs. Taking time for telephone conversations or conferences with these other members of the helping professions pays dividends.

TERMS FREQUENTLY USED IN MEDICAL REPORTS

Alexia. Visual aphasia or word blindness; inability to read because of a brain lesion.

Anoxia. Oxygen deficiency or lack.

Aphasia. Defect or loss of the power of expression by speech, writing, or signs, or of comprehending spoken or written language, because of injury to or disease of the brain centers. *Expressive aphasia.* Inability to speak or write. *Global aphasia.* Total aphasia. *Receptive aphasia.* Inability to understand or to read.

Apraxia. Loss of ability to perform purposeful movements, without paralysis of the parts concerned.

Aprophoria. Inability to express articulated words in speech or writing.

Arteriosclerosis. A condition marked by loss of elasticity, and by thickening and hardening, of the arteries. *Generalized arteriosclerosis* (*G.A.S.*). Widespread arteriosclerosis; term often used to indicate cerebral arteriosclerosis or senility.

Atherosclerosis. A form of arteriosclerosis in which the inner lining of a blood vessel is chiefly involved; fatty masses developing and hardening to clog the vessels—"rust in the pipes."

Carotid. The principal arteries of the neck.

Cerebral anemia. Deficient blood supply to the brain.

Cerebral hemorrhage. Apoplexy, or rupture of a cerebral blood vessel.

Cerebral ischemia. Deficiency of blood supply to the brain.

Cerebral necrosis. Death of brain tissue; term occasionally used to denote dementia or senility.

Cerebral thrombosis. The formation of a clot in the wall of a cerebral artery producing an occlusion or blocking of the vessel.

Cerebral vascular accident. "Stroke" or **CVA**.

Chronic brain syndrome. Brain damage from various causes, including psychosis and head injury, and resulting in a behavior pattern characterized by confusion, forgetfulness, poor judgment, and other features similar to those of senility.

Cortical atrophy. Wasting and death of the cortex of the brain; term often used to denote mental deficiency.

Dicumarol. A drug used to prevent blood from clotting in the vessels.

Disuse atrophy. Muscle wasting caused by lack of use of the part.

Dysarthria. Imperfect articulation in speech.

Encephalomalacia. Softening of the brain.

Flaccid. Describing a limp form of paralysis.

Heparin. A drug similar to dicumarol in purpose.

Hemiparesis. Partial paralysis of half of body; term sometimes used synonymously with *hemiplegia*.

Hemiplegia. Paralysis of half the body.

Homonymous hemianopsia. An eye condition usually resulting from a cerebral vascular accident in which there is blindness of one eye toward the nose and in the other in the half toward the temple.

Infarction. Death of tissue.

Intracranial. Within the cranium.

Monoplegia. Paralysis of one limb.

Necrosis. Death of a cell or of a group of cells surrounded by living tissue.

Occlusion. Clogging by a clot or thrombosis; state of being closed.

Papilledema. Choked disc of the eye; optic neuritis caused by intracranial pressure.

Spastic. Describes a tightened muscular condition.

Vasospasm. Spasm of the blood vessels, resulting in decrease in their caliber.

Vasodilatation. Dilation of a blood vessel.

CHAPTER XIII

Cancer

CANCER, the second highest cause of death, is predominantly a disease of persons more than forty years of age, and increases in incidence with advancing age. Whereas the disease is of special concern to those who are working with the aged and disabled, all social workers need to be informed about cancer because no age group is immune. Curiously enough, cancer now causes more deaths among children under fifteen than any other disease, largely because the other diseases have been brought under control.

Approximately one-third of those who have cancer are cured. Even though we tend to think of the disease in terms of its fatality, many patients live for a long time. This period should be made as comfortable and satisfying as possible. The public assistance worker's contribution to the meaningfulness of these months or years is more substantial than is commonly realized. It may be difficult to inculcate in ourselves an objective approach, but obviously the cancer patient merits the same intelligent consideration of his needs as any other.

Great strides have been made in the medical management of cancer during the past several years. Substantial relief of pain and other distressing symptoms is now possible in most cases in which the patient is given the benefit of skilled and thoughtful medical supervision. Although it is emotionally difficult to work with clients who we know are going to die, we need not feel that visits mean witnessing intolerable suffering about which nothing can be done. Both the client and the worker can, therefore, feel more free to consider the client's normal human needs as well as the difficult problems posed by the disease.

General Medical Base for Social Planning

CAUSE

The cause of cancer is still unknown. It is neither infectious nor inherited, although family susceptibility seems to be established. Certain cells start to multiply rapidly and in a disorderly manner. Although the basic cause is still beyond the ken of science, there are well-supported theories about some of the secondary or exciting causes. Hormonal changes are believed to influence the growth of the potentially lawless cells. Chemicals, as in aniline dyes and soot, may be cancer-inciting, as may also be overexposure to X rays or to the sun. Repeated irritation may also be causative. Further, certain precancerous conditions exist including certain moles, chronic ulcers, and chronic infection.

There are sex differences in the incidence and mortality from cancer. Men, for example, are prone to cancer of the lung, stomach, mouth, bladder, and prostate; women are most likely to have cancers of the breast, uterus, and intestines. In some parts of the body, as in the blood stream and in the rectum, the mortality rates and incidence are not far apart in the two sexes. The over-all death rate is somewhat, though not markedly, greater in men.

There are two broad groups of cancers: *carcinomas,* or those arising in *epithelial* (covering or lining) tissue; and *sarcomas,* or those arising in connective or supporting tissue, as in bones, fat, lymph and blood vessels. The technical names of cancers describe the kind: for example, "adeno-*carcinoma*" or "lympho*sarcoma.*" Medical reports frequently merely use the terms "carcinoma" (abbreviated as CA) and "sarcoma."

DEVELOPMENT

A cancer is a malignant tumor. It is distinguished from harmless (benign) tumors by the fact that whereas the benign tumor merely grows and stays in one place, usually surrounded by a membrane, the malignant or cancerous tumor invades surrounding tissue, destroying normal adjacent cells as it grows. Further, it tends to spread to distant parts of the body.

Cancer cells, if not removed early enough, may get into the blood stream or lymph channels, or be dislodged into other organs and start new growths (*metastases*). Once the disease has *metastasized,* it is incurable. This fact explains why there is such emphasis upon early detection and treatment, and why surgery needs to take in a wide surrounding area to include all cancer cells and to avoid the possibility of dislodging them.

ONSET AND SYMPTOMS

Onset is frequently insidious, producing such vague or minor symptoms in the early stages that the individual either does not know anything is wrong or hesitates to go to a doctor.

If he does, the doctor may not detect anything. For this reason the private cancer societies vigorously attempt to educate the public and the medical profession to investigate symptoms which may be suspicious and which everyone is expected to recognize: lumps, bleeding, hoarseness, persistent indigestion, white patches, and unexplained fatigue or sudden weight loss. Health education can backfire and cause unnecessary fear and consequent procrastination in seeing a doctor.

Because symptoms are so often nonexistent or minor, early detection of cancer is often dependent on deliberate measures such as periodic health examination, routine monthly breast palpation, mass chest X rays, and the physician's use of techniques to secure cell examinations. Once the cancer is detected, it may be eradicated. If it is not, the wild cells continue their growth at a greatly variable rate until they have destroyed the functioning of vital tissue and death results.

FACTORS AFFECTING LIFE EXPECTANCY

The social worker should learn from the physician how fast growing a malignant tumor is and whether it has metastasized by the time it is found. The rate of growth varies greatly. The older a person is, the slower all his cells grow, so that ordinarily the life expectancy of an old person with cancer is much longer than that of a young person. For example, leukemia is rapidly fatal in a child, but the form which older persons have may permit them to live for many years.

Some cancers, whatever age the person is, are swift, and others slow. For example, a *basal cell carcinoma* of the skin is slow and easy to control, whereas the dread *malignant melanoma,* which develops from a dark mole, is exceedingly swift. Social workers cannot be expected to memorize and to retain the technical names of the fast- and slow-growing cancers, but, as will be emphasized later, it is important to find out from the doctor about the rate of growth in order to have a sound base for social planning.

For practical reasons, the accessibility of the cancer is one of the major determinants in life expectancy. If it is visible, as on the skin or in a body orifice, where the symptoms will be apparent and the doctor can examine it, early detection and removal are facilitated. Mortality rates vary greatly according to site—skin cancer, for example, causing few fatalities, whereas stomach, intestinal, and lung cancer cause many deaths.

Life expectancy is affected by the amenability of the tumor to the delaying action of palliative measures, as well as by the possibility of complete eradication.

Medical discoveries are uneven. Certain treatments will create a temporary slowing of some kinds of tumors but not of others. For example, cancer of the reproductive organs can be slowed down by sex hormones. Male hormones (*androgens*) prove effective for some uterine and breast cancers of women of child-bearing age; female hormones (*estrogens*) are effective for cancers of the prostate. Certain chemicals, notably nitrogen mustard, have been found effective in slowing down leukemia or blood cancer and also lung cancer. The male hormone (*testosterone*) is also said to be effective in treating bone cancer.

Radiation by X ray or radium is effective in shrinking the size of many cancers, especially those of the breast, thyroid, prostate, and lymph glands. Radioisotopes, from the waste of atomic piles, are being used in treatment centers that have the facilities to handle them. At this early stage of development of the peaceful use of the atom, these radioisotopes are largely limited to radioactive cobalt, radioactive iodine for thyroid cancer, and radioactive phosphorus for some blood cancers.

The amount of action in the part of the body involved is also a vital factor in determining life expectancy. Some organs, like the lungs or intestines, are constantly expanding and contracting. Women's breasts and uteri during the reproductive period and during periods of hormonal changes, as in the menopause, are subject to many physiological changes. Thus, cancer cells are easily dislodged or thrown off into the blood stream to create new sites for themselves and to add greatly to the difficulty of eradication.

TREATMENT

Treatment should be immediate upon discovery, to avoid any further possibility of metastasis. The client's life often depends not only upon timing but upon the competence of the surgeon, so that the best available skill should be sought. Surgery, deep X ray, radium, and radioisotopes offer the only effective means of treatment at the present time. Salves and diets are quackery.

Surgery is frequently combined with X-ray therapy, either before or after the operation. Doctors disagree about X-ray treatment. Some types of cancer respond well to radiation, and others do not. X-ray therapy causes substantial discomfort. An amount large enough to cure may irritate the skin, with resulting rash or blisters over a period of weeks. This must be properly taken care of under nursing or medical direction.

Nausea, weakness, and loss of appetite are usual results of the tissue destruction caused by X-ray therapy. The symptoms are severe enough to interfere with the client's use of public transportation and usual household activities. Deep X ray to the abdomen may further cause the inconvenience of diarrhea and difficulty in urination. X-ray treatment of the pelvis causes artificial menopause but does not interfere with sexual response.

Surgery must be extensive or "radical," as mentioned earlier, in order to avoid the danger of cutting into or dislodging any outlying cancer cells. Because most cancer patients are older persons, there is considerable debate about the advisability of operating. The risks are greater, and some professional persons hold to the theory that the older patient should be allowed a shorter time to live without going through the pain and disfigurement of surgery.

However, others feel that old persons deserve a chance to live just as much as the young, and should not be deprived of what surgery has to offer. Modern operating techniques have greatly reduced the risk to older persons, so that unless the client has major heart trouble or his condition has seriously deteriorated before surgery, the element of risk from age alone is considered small.

Reactions to surgery vary according to its extent, the meaning the loss has to the particular patient, his temperament, and according to the doctor's preparation of the patient and to postsurgical management. Most persons would prefer to lose an arm or a leg and live a longer life; most can learn to take care of a colostomy (an artificial opening made in the abdomen for discharge of feces) after surgery for cancer of the colon or rectum. Each person attaches his own significance to loss of body parts. Some reactions are readily understood—for example, the feeling of a young married woman about the loss of a breast. Some reactions seem illogical to the outsider, but are as valid to the person concerned.

Cancer of the head and neck often leads to extremely radical surgery, resulting at times in loss of speech through removal of the larynx or tongue, interference with the ability to swallow normally, or in loss of parts of the face. No one can accept such consequences with equanimity, especially if the physician has failed to give details of the consequences before the operation. These patients deserve our maximum effort in arranging comfort, care, and moral support.

Radium and radioisotope therapy operate on the same principle as X-ray treatment, the rays destroying the cancer cells and their ability to multiply. Radium is implanted in solid organs in platinum needles, or is placed inside hollow organs in capsules. Its advantage over X ray is that the rays do not have to go through and thus destroy so much normal tissue to reach the organ; its disadvantages are that it requires great skill to administer properly, being dangerous otherwise, and is usually available only in certain large treatment centers.

Radioisotope treatment has the advantage of being painless and simple from the patient's viewpoint. The tasteless isotope is swallowed in a glass of water, and later checked by a Geiger counter. It is, however, a dangerous and highly complex tool to use, and is as yet limited in application. The treatment operates on the principle that certain isotopes select only certain kinds of tissues in which to lodge —for example, radioactive iodine in thyroid tissue only. This isotope is valuable in spotting metastases if the tumor has started to grow in remote places; these extensions will also frequently pick up the isotope, so that their radioactive presence can be detected with the Geiger counter.

PALLIATIVE MEASURES

The fear of cancer seems the result less of the fear of death than of fear of intolerable pain. Fortunately, in this area much progress has been made. Extreme unmanageable pain is inevitable only in the terminal phases of some cancers, such as those of the brain, face, rectum, bladder, or female genital organs, provided that the physician is sufficiently knowledgeable and concerned to apply all the known modern methods of palliation, and provided that environmental measures are undertaken which are in the zealous social worker's reach. It is authoritatively stated that in most instances life can be made at least tolerable even in far advanced cancer, if serious effort is made. Too often, in ignorance, we assume that the cancer patient must undergo untold misery, and fail to raise the question with the physician as to what can be done.

In addition to the initial operation attempting to eradicate the cancer, various surgical measures can be undertaken later which bring relief from nausea or pain and prolong life. New tumors may be removed; relief from the symptoms of intestinal obstruction may be secured by "short circuit" operations which take out diseased parts and join healthy parts together (*anastomosis*); plastic tubes can be implanted and artificial openings made which overcome dangers of starvation or other difficulties. In extreme cases, nerve-cutting operations which produce paralysis but stop pain may be resorted to.

Further examples of treatment include: X-ray treatment of metastases, which shrink size and reduce pressure on adjacent organs and nerves; hormone therapy, which slows down prostate and female reproductive organ cancers; testosterone therapy, which reduces the danger of fractures where bone metastases exist; the use of nitrogen mustard in certain selected cases. Some palliative measures bring their own discomforts, notably X-ray therapy and testosterone. The latter causes masculine distribution of hair, deepening of voice, and increased libido which some women find distressing.

The so-called "general supportive measures" are of especial interest to social workers. To combat weakness, weight loss, anemia, debility, and loss of morale, and to keep the patient up and about and as cheerful as possible—in other words, to extend his period of useful life and shorten the period of misery and dependence—blood transfusions, tranquilizers, and body-building medicines are often prescribed.

Keeping wounds clean reduces the odors that are difficult for patients and their family and associates to endure and, therefore, boosts morale. This often involves irrigations that the public health nurse can perform or teach the family to carry out. Artificial openings for breathing, eating, and elimination require medical supplies and attention under skilled supervision. Every advanced cancer patient should have instruction and help from a nurse, either from a clinic or from the public health department.

Diet which caters to the palate and, which in head, neck, stomach, and intestinal cancer, is suited to impaired eating or digestive functions, is of great importance in avoiding debility, unnecessary discomfort, and lowered morale. The guidance of a nurse in these matters, as well as the experience of the patient and his family, is helpful if a busy doctor has not had the time to prescribe in detail.

Narcotics prove effective in relieving all but the worst pain if they are alternated and prescribed judiciously. Occasionally there is fear of addiction, on the part of either patient or doctor, which is illogical in light of the circumstances. Withholding drugs from a cancer patient must be faced for what it is—cruelty. Fortunately, most physicians prescribe narcotics and are able to circumvent patients' objections by using kindly deceits.

SHOULD THE PATIENT BE TOLD?

Doctors differ in their attitude toward this most difficult question, but experienced physicians usually spare their patients the weight of inevitable despair over impending death, gauging their comments by the manner in which the patient indicates what he wants to know. Although most persons who have not faced critical illness say that they would want to be told, few actually can live with equanimity unless they hold on to some hope that matters are not so bad as they fear. When patients ask their doctors, "Is there nothing that can be done for me?" they have in mind abandonment to intolerable pain. As the doctor can truthfully reassure them on this point, his usual answer is that he can, of course, help.

Information on life and death must be given by the physician and by no one else. This matter of ethics is basic.

Since the course and implications of cancer in different parts of the body vary considerably, the following detail is presented about cancer of the lung, uterus, intestine, and leukemia.

CANCER OF THE LUNG

Cancer of the lung is the leading cause of mortality from cancer in men. Its rapid increase and poor prognosis create cause for much concern. The disease is at least five times more common in men than in women, and is especially prevalent in men of more than forty-five years of age. Heavy smoking and other causes of chronic irritation are now considered to be definitely contributory to its development.

There are three main types of cancer of the lung, and each has a characteristic rate of growth, set of symptoms, and tendency to metastasize. The symptoms vary according to the type and the location in the lung. Often there are no symptoms in the early stage, which is one of the main reasons the prognosis is so poor.

Routine chest X rays and cell studies offer the best hope for early detection. Diagnosis sometimes cannot be made except by surgery and pathological examination of affected tissue. When delayed symptoms develop, they frequently include coughing and wheezing, and sometimes other signs such as pain in the chest, blood-streaked sputum, swelling in the neck, and shortness of breath, and, in the late stages, anemia, weight loss, and debility.

Surgery for removal of the lobe of the lung or of the whole lung is performed if the cancer is detected before it has extended to surrounding areas or has metastasized. X-ray therapy is occasionally used curatively, and frequently used palliatively. Nitrogen mustard is also used palliatively at times.

The percentage of five-year cures or even three-year cures is very small, and death may occur from three to six months after symptoms appear. Consequently, in lung cancers, planning usually needs to concern itself with securing the greatest possible relief and comfort for the patient, and with anticipation of family interruption in a relatively short period of time.

CANCER OF THE UTERUS

Cancer of the uterus has a much more hopeful outlook, with about 40 per cent of the patients achieving five-year cures. It is most frequently located in the cervix or the opening of the uterus. However, especially in older women who have not borne children, it may occur in the lining of the body of the uterus (*corpus uteri*).

Cancer of the cervix is one of the most frequently found, occurring primarily in women who have had more than one child, and most often during the menopausal period. A silent or noninvasive stage has been identified, during which time the cancer cells can be detected through the well-known and painless "Pap" smear technique used by the doctor and laboratory at the time of pelvic examination.

Cancer of the cervix does not tend to metastasize early, so that if either the silent stage or early carcinoma is identified during routine physical examination, effective early treatment can be instituted. This, obviously, is the reason why routine pelvic examinations are so desirable for women between thirty and sixty years of age. If cancer is detected and treated in the silent stage, there is 100 per cent cure.

Symptoms, unfortunately, are frequently shrugged off or not recognized as needing attention, for they resemble menstrual irregularity. Occasional spotting, watery discharge, irregular bleeding, and lengthening of the menstrual periods are the usual early signs. Bleeding after menopause is a most urgent sign, but even among the health-educated, the tendency is to avoid the unpleasantness of a pelvic examination by rationalizing it as a delayed menstrual period.

If carcinoma of the cervix is discovered while it is still in early stages, before it has spread to the pelvic wall, approved treatment consists of either a very extensive pelvic operation (*radical panhysterectomy*), or combined radium and X-ray treatment. Because of the risks of the surgery, irradiation is considered preferable by some authorities. Good results are achieved (about 25 per cent of the cases having five-year cures), when the treatment is carried out by skilled physicians with good facilities. Convalescence is uncomfortable and weakness prolonged after either procedure.

If the cancer is not discovered and treated until it has extended to surrounding organs, it cannot be treated surgically. X-ray therapy is used for palliation. Hormones are no longer considered helpful. Severe complications result especially from damage to the uterus and bladder, with death usually occurring from these complications. The terminal phase of cancer of the cervix is characterized by intractable pain, a matter which has implications for the social as well as the medical planning involved. Clients with far-advanced cancer of the cervix need our most extensive efforts.

Cancer of the body of the uterus is much less common, and is a slow-growing tumor found primarily in women in their sixties who have not had children. It tends to metastasize, but if detected early enough and the patient's condition permits the surgery necessary, the prognosis is among the best for all cancers—the very best, in fact, for cancer of an internal organ.

This type of growth starts in the lining (*endometrium*), and is said to be frequently antedated by polyps or benign growths. Hysterectomy for this condition is a common precaution. Symptoms of cancer include a watery discharge, pain, postmenopausal bleeding, or sometimes constipation or urinary symptoms.

Because the older age of women who have this type of cancer with the accompaniments of age, such as hypertension or diabetes, often makes the very radical operation inadvisable, treatment may be by a combination of radium and surgery or radium and X ray.

If the treatment is begun too late, the cancer spreads to surrounding lymph nodes, and sometimes to brain, lungs, or elsewhere. Palliative measures include hormones, X ray, and the general supportive measures described earlier. Length of life is dependent upon the response to palliation and upon the site of metastases and their effects.

Women with cancer of the uterus who have not had treatment in time present complicated nursing problems, partly owing to infections which are secondary to the disease and to the prevalence of involvement of organs of elimination, and also because of pain. The good prognosis of early cases makes clear the importance of helping clients take advantage of detection and early treatment measures.

CANCER OF THE INTESTINE

The intestine is one of the most common sites of cancer in both men and women, though it occurs more frequently in men. Most of these carcinomas are situated in the large bowel, including the colon and rectum. Of the operable cases (about 60 per cent) one-third to one-half receive five-year cures, which is considered a good prognosis for the group as a whole.

There are three types of cancer, all adenocarcinomas, with varying characteristics and sites. The symptoms vary accordingly but in general consist in the early stages of minor changes in bowel habits such as constipation and/or diarrhea, bloating, mild colicky pain, mucus or blood in the stools, or loss of appetite. Because the early symptoms resemble those of minor gastric upsets, they are often ignored. Blood may be thought to be caused by hemorrhoids. Not until bleeding, obvious masses in the abdomen, or distressing symptoms of obstruction develop do many persons seek medical attention. Symptoms may include severe anemia or may resemble the symptoms of appendicitis.

Necessary tests to establish the diagnosis involve uncomfortable procedures including barium enemas followed by X ray and proctoscopic or sigmoidoscopic examinations. The latter are sometimes painful, often creating reluctance in the patient to continue with medical care. Treatment is by surgery, the kind depending on where the tumor is and how large it is. Preparation for surgery requires several days in the hospital, and the operation itself may carry considerable risk, necessitating major skill and good nursing care. Convalescence is frequently painful and debility prolonged.

Cancers of the lower sigmoid and rectum usually require a permanent colostomy mentioned before as a measure after which the bowel discharges through an opening made in the abdomen. Colostomy bags may be necessary, and the patient may need to be taught to regulate evacuation by means of irrigations and diet.

The patient is taught the care of the colostomy in the hospital. Irrigations are time-consuming and unpleasant at best, and some patients find the mutilation and the revulsion such severe psychic upsets that they are slow and resistive in learning how to give themselves the necessary care.

The necessary changes in diet to avoid roughage and gas also create problems familiar to social workers. However, successful colostomy regulation is important in facilitating the patient's future work and social contacts and, therefore, his feelings about himself and his condition.

When cancer of the intestine has progressed beyond the curatively operable stage before discovery, palliative surgery may sometimes be performed to relieve obstructions and thus lessen pain and nausea. Nausea and retching are among the most intolerable burdens of advanced cancer, so that it is fortunate that suction apparatus, certain drugs and sedatives, and some surgery have a great deal to offer in reducing the patient's burden. Length of life is, as in other types of cancer, dependent upon the site and damage of metastases as well as upon the rate and place of growth of the original tumor.

LEUKEMIA

Leukemia is the most common blood cancer, and accounts for about 4 per cent of all cancer deaths. It is more common in men than in women. The disease is one in which white-cell manufacture is greatly increased; these cells penetrate the various tissues of the body, especially the liver, spleen, bone marrow, and lymph nodes. There are a number of varieties of leukemia, the common forms being *granulocytic* and *lymphocytic,* referring to type of cells involved, and each may be *acute, subacute,* or *chronic.*

The differentiations into acute or chronic are the important terms for social workers to remember, for these have to do with the course and prognosis.

Acute leukemia occurs most frequently in persons of less than twenty-five years of age, mostly in children of less than five, but may occasionally exist in older persons. It runs a rapid course, with high fever, hemorrhages, and death occurring within from a few months to a year or two. Repeated blood transfusions, certain medicines, and the steroids—ACTH and cortisone—are used for treatment, sometimes creating pronounced abatement for several months but not achieving cures.

The chronic leukemias usually develop during the decades of middle life. In young persons the expectancy is limited to two to five years, but older persons may live for five or ten years or, in a few instances, considerably longer. The disease is characterized by flare-ups and abatement (*exacerbations* and *remissions*) the periods of abatement in chronic lymphocytic leukemia sometimes lasting for long periods of time. The chronic lymphocytic type of leukemia ordinarily occurs in the forty- to sixty-year age group.

Chronic leukemia has a slow gradual onset, with weakness, fatigue, loss of weight, and poor color as early signs. There may be fever and chills, shortness of breath, and palpitations from the developing severe anemia; enlargement of the liver and spleen (*hepatomegaly* and *splenomegaly*) and lymph nodes occurs. There may be also an abnormal tendency to bleed. The laboratory evidence of anemia and increased white-cell or leukocyte count further informs the doctor of the diagnosis. As the disease progresses, increasing weakness and additional symptoms occur depending on the tissues invaded.

Treatment is not directed toward cure but rather toward relief of symptoms and prolongation of life. X-ray therapy, either over the entire body or of the spleen, is most common; antibiotics, blood transfusions, and sometimes radioactive phosphorus (P32) or nitrogen mustard are also used. A number of chemotherapeutic agents are being developed and utilized.

Respiratory infections and hemorrhages cause complications and must be guarded against through dieting and other measures to increase general resistance, morale, and avoidance of falls or other trauma.

Other, less frequent, blood cancers related to leukemia include *Hodgkin's disease* and *lymphosarcoma*. There are also malignant blood diseases of the reverse order, in which the manufacture of red rather than white blood cells occur —for example, *polycythemia vera*. Each of these has its own characteristics and usual course, the common factor being the lack at this time of any cure, with the notable exception of *lymphosarcoma* which is sometimes cured by X-ray therapy or by surgery.

Implications for Public Assistance

THE WORKER'S ATTITUDE

It is no disgrace to feel so uncomfortable in the presence of a sick person that one cannot work constructively with him. Deep-rooted feelings about cancer are relatively common in professional persons, social workers, clergymen, and —surprisingly enough—even in some doctors. The worker needs to undertake a frank examination of her own personal attitudes, and, if an immobilizing or overwhelming fear or repugnance exists, an arrangement for others to provide the services the client needs.

The supervisor may be able to transfer the case to another worker; if this cannot be done, the worker may be able to find a nurse, a clergyman, or a volunteer to take responsibility for many of the services to the client. It is important that the worker not disguise her own feelings to herself and then procrastinate or find reasons for not seeing the client or fail to do those things the client needs to have done for him.

However, before giving up on one's own attitudes, it is well to break them up in parts and analyze just what it is that is causing the discomfort. Is it the fear of or knowledge of the client's fatal diagnosis? If so, do we know that the client is going to die, and, in fact, any sooner than anyone else? If it is the eventual fatality that is bothering us, are we afraid that the client is going to pour out his despair and that we will have no answer or no way of comforting him? Or are we just afraid we could not bear to witness his emotion?

If this is what we find to be troubling us, we can reassure ourselves on a good many points. The chances are that the client's death is not imminent, and that even if it is, he is concerned with many urgent matters of living, considerations of the moment and the day, which he wants to talk with us about. By relieving the client of worries that are within our scope, we are being useful to him and contributing toward his well-being. As we involve ourselves in these problems that have to be solved, our own emotions get pushed back into proper perspective.

In most instances, persons prefer not to talk about fatality even to close relatives or friends because they cannot bear to. They often use such a good pretense of not knowing their condition that it is difficult to tell just what they do know or suspect. In these cases, the worker can only "play the game" the way the client wants it, never breaking through his defenses but dealing with situations "until he gets better" and using whatever terms for the disease he uses. If the client does ask questions about his condition, the only response the worker can make is to suggest that he ask the doctor, and, if necessary, to arrange for him to see the doctor.

If, however, the client does have the kind of relationship with us that permits him to use us to bring out his feelings about impending death, which is relatively rare, we have been paid a high compliment and have been given an unusual opportunity to be of service. Death means many different things to different people; humanity has various kinds of fears.

One person may be concerned about what will happen to the family, and this is within our scope to help with; one may be concerned about life after death, and this calls for finding a clergyman to discuss the matter with the client; one may be worried about burial arrangements, and here again we can normally be helpful; another may be in great anxiety about future medical care or for relief of pain, and here we can be helpful by calling on the doctor and the nurse. In other words, even the experience of fearing death is broken down into parts in most human experience. By dealing with the part, we ourselves can handle it, and can then be of great assistance to the client in reducing it to a size he himself can handle.

Probably the most common reason for immobilizing anxiety within ourselves is the fear of seeing and hearing great distress. Because it is in the area of palliation that the strides have been made in cancer management, the client who is under good care is not going to be in intolerable distress until the last, when he will probably be in the hospital and not accessible for interview. If by chance we discover a client who is at home or in an out-of-home care facility and who is in pain or needs help of a physical nature, then it is well that the client's need is discovered so that proper medical and/or nursing care can be arranged quickly.

If in spite of these things we find we are unable to deal with our emotions, and we find ourselves procrastinating in helping the client with cancer, we must accept this limitation as we do any other problem, and create ways to see that the client is served by someone else.

SPECIAL NEEDS

In the foregoing discussion of our own feelings, it was mentioned that the client usually wants to talk with us and to secure our help with the problems of living rather than those of dying. In addition to basic needs, the chances are that he will have special material needs, in connection with desirable living arrangements, diet, transportation, medical supplies, laundry, bedding, and/or attendant cares. Earlier mention has been made of the importance of general supportive measures of a social nature which keep the client up and about and as cheerful as possible. When weakness makes the bed important to the client, the state of the mattress and bedding and facilities for laundry need to be explored if the client remains at home. What is desirable will be predicated on an understanding of the recipient's individual medical situation and prognosis.

USE AND COÖRDINATION OF HUMAN RESOURCES

In earlier chapters it has been brought out that contrary to our usual assumption that the client is the best source of information, the client is not a good source in regard to his medical condition. Especially when a grave diagnosis exists, the doctor is not likely to have shared fully with the patient, and the client can be expected to have distorted ideas resulting from his own reactions to what he does know so far.

Securing necessary medical information from the physician may be complicated by several factors, but made easier than usual by others. The physician may be afraid to give information to the social worker for fear she will reveal it to the client; he may not know the exact prognosis and may dislike to be "put behind the eight ball"; occasionally, he may be one of those sensitive and awkward physicians who find it difficult not to be able to cure their patients and who defend themselves against their feelings by ignoring the patient or brushing off questions.

Social workers do encounter occasional physicians who are busy and who do not want to be bothered by welfare clients. However, in general, the client with the grave diagnosis receives the most thoughtful medical attention. The doctor is worried about the client, sympathetic toward him, and is grateful that a conscientious social worker is available to coöperate with him in the client's behalf.

When the client is under private care and not in an institution, the social worker can avoid the problems and capitalize on the assets by going to the doctor's office to talk with him. (He probably will not put much on a medical report for fear the information will get back to the client.) At that time, the worker will want to know whether the cancer was discovered early enough to be eradicated in all probability, or whether it has already metastasized or become inoperable; if the latter, what kind of palliative measures are recommended and approximately how long the client will live if this can be determined.

The social worker will want to know whether hospitalization or nursing-home care is to be expected soon; if hospitalization, whether it will be for the terminal period or merely for palliative work. The social worker can find out from the doctor what will be important in keeping the client comfortable and active at home as long as possible.

It is important to find out how much the doctor has told the client and how much he thinks the client suspects, so that the worker can gauge her interviews accordingly without revealing any information. Further, she will want to make sure that some responsible family member knows the client's medical situation and, if the doctor has not talked to a member of the family, to arrange with him and the family member so that they can talk.

Frequently, more than one conference with the doctor will be necessary as the client's situation changes. If a good relationship has been established at the time of the initial visit, further information can often be secured by telephone.

The fact that clients with cancer have usually been hospital patients means that most of them will have been in a county hospital and may be dependent on the clinic for supervision. Thus, the medical worker will be available in some cases to secure the kind of information that is needed, or arrange a three-way conference with the doctor. Here, again, the gravity of the diagnosis is an asset, for exceptions are often made to usual routines in order to permit maximum benefit to the gravely ill client and his family.

The client who was a county hospital patient and is under clinic care may be in special need of the social worker's alertness to his condition. If he has an anxious, articulate family, he probably is in no danger of being lost to sight; but if he is alone or if the family is handicapped by language or apathetic resignation to circumstances, the homebound client may be neglected until the public assistance worker takes initiative in getting him back under active care. The turnover in intern and resident staff at the county hospital, the great pressure of work, and the impersonality of big clinics make it important that the weak or sick person at home or in an out-of-home care facility have someone who will act for him.

The public health or visiting nurse has been mentioned as an invaluable resource for the client with cancer. Some counties which are limited in public health nursing staff assign the nurses only to special clinics such as tuberculosis; but, again, the gravity of the diagnosis usually comes to the cancer patient's aid when the social worker makes a special request for help to a given client. The public health nurse does not usually give bedside care, but she does help the client and family set up the supplies and equipment they need and makes sure that someone is taught how to give irrigations, take care of dressings, prepare special foods, bathe a bed patient, and so on. Further, she knows how to describe the client's condition to the doctor in a way that is most meaningful to him.

Clergymen have a great deal to offer to sick people. When a person is confronted with catastrophe or life-threatening experiences, he is forced to face vital issues that may be otherwise obscured by the clutter and complacency of normal living. The active church member will ordinarily make his own arrangements, but the many clients without church ties or who have been a long time away from old church ties may greatly welcome a visit and sometimes a developing relationship with a clergyman.

The choice of a clergyman is important if the client does not have his own. One begins with the main divisions of religion, choosing a priest for a Catholic, a fundamentalist Protestant for a Protestant whose old ties were with a fundamentalist church, and so on. If the community is large enough, the worker attempts within this framework to find a clergyman known to be compassionate, able to give the time, and psychologically capable of working with sick people. Experience with a given minister is the best gauge, or the county hospital worker or the public health nurse may be able to make good suggestions.

Leading into the subject of having a minister call needs to be handled carefully. The best approach is to ask the client whether he would like to have a certain clergyman call. This can be done, for example, after the client has been voicing discouragement, or in response to some comment or question which shows that the client is groping philosophically.

The full use of human resources within the community is suggested not only because the problem merits and because time is saved thereby, but because medical, nursing, and theological areas are outside the competence of the social worker. To attempt to deal with any one of them alone leads to entangling relationships and inadequate services to the client. These resources can include such private health agencies as the American Cancer Society, which supplies dressings and, in some communities, occasional financial help toward attendant care and friendly visiting.

PLACEMENT

Should the client stay home? This question usually arises sooner or later. The elements which go into the decision are: whether necessary pain-relieving and nursing procedures can be carried on at home; what do the client and his family want; what kinds of facilities are available; and what is the effect of the client's condition upon the family, especially on children and on the caretaker.

Organized home care programs have shown that clients can be adequately cared for at home and are happier even in relatively poor surroundings if the physician is willing to come to the home as often as necessary if there are available nursing services, and if the family is willing to undergo the necessary sacrifices. Because they know that the end is in sight, families can more frequently bear the burden of care of a cancer patient than they can of a relative whose prognosis is indeterminate. Clients themselves are almost always happier and better off at home, unless they cannot get the medicine and specialized help they need there.

PLANNING FOR THE FAMILY

Planning for the children after her death is ordinarily the greatest concern of a mother who knows she has cancer or of anyone responsible for dependents. The client may lead obliquely into the matter rather than asking the worker's help directly. It is better to wait for the client to touch on the subject than to initiate it.

The worker should give the client opportunity to talk about the children or the dependents, and be sensitive to indications that he is showing anxiety and wants to talk about the future. Often it is possible to reassure her that "if anything should happen" the children would be placed in good homes, or would be sent to relatives, or could be kept together. It is important to convey that the worker will be standing by and will take responsibility if there are no relatives with whom the mother has already made arrangements or if she indicates she is not sure she could put trust in them.

The fact that the client needs the framework of a relationship and opportunities to talk when he is ready is one of the reasons why either the worker or some professional person other than the doctor should see the client regularly. If children are old enough to understand or to fear, they too need the support of knowing a helping person is available in advance of the time when placement is necessary or advisable, which is usually in advance of the client's actual death. The children's welfare is always a consideration to be weighed in home care of a client with terminal disease; needless to say, they should be spared the trauma of witnessing untoward events or the client's acute distress.

COUNSELING

In early or suspected cancer, the listening, supporting, and counseling role of the social worker may assume lifesaving importance. Postponement of medical examinations or treatment is common, often because of fear of what will be discovered or recommended. Emotional support from a friendly, understanding person often enables a frightened person to take a step he dreads. Misapprehensions exist that can often be cleared up by finding out first what it is that the client is afraid of, and then securing accurate information and relaying it to the client, or preferably arranging for a conference between the client and the physician, or asking a nurse to talk with the client. Arguments and impasses obviously should be avoided.

Decisions about operations must be made by the client. Social workers can help by giving emotional support, by clarifying information, and by simplifying arrangements, but active persuasion is contraindicated. The risk of surgery is real, and only the patient can take the responsibility of decision. The role of the worker is essentially one of being sure that the patient has the facts on which to weigh his decision, that he is not confused by irrational fears or left alone emotionally when he is confronted by a very difficult task, and that the social factors in his situation do not constitute obstacles to his care.

TERMS FREQUENTLY USED IN MEDICAL REPORTS

Adenoma. A harmless or benign tumor.

Androgen. Male hormone.

Basal cell. One of the cells of the deep layer of the skin; the name given to one type of skin cancer.

Benign. Not malignant or recurrent; favorable for recovery.

Biopsy. Diagnostic examination of a piece of tissue removed from a living subject.

Carcinoma. A malignant growth tending to infiltrate the surrounding tissues and giving rise to metastases; scientific name for one general type of cancer.

Colostomy. Technically, the operation for forming an artificial opening into the colon; in common usage, an opening in the abdomen for the discharge of feces.

Endometrial. The mucous membrane that lines the cavity of the uterus.

Epithelium. The covering of the skin and of mucous membranes.

Estrogen. A commercial ovarian extract or female hormone.

Gastrostomy. The operation of forming an opening into the stomach.

Hodgkin's disease. Form of lymph-node cancer.

Leukemia. A malignant disease of the blood-forming organs; cancer of the blood.

Leukocyte. A colorless cell mass, such as a white blood corpuscle, pus corpuscle.

Lymphosarcoma. A malignant tumor arising in lymph tissue.

Malignant. A virulent tumor; a cancer.

Metastasis. The transfer of malignant cells from one organ or part to another.

Myeloma. A malignant tumor composed of cells of a type resembling cells often found in the bone marrow.

Neoplasm. Any new and abnormal growth such as a tumor.

Papanicolaou stain ("Pap" smear). A method of detecting the presence of malignant cells by the examination of cells shed in body cavities or in fluids.

Papillary adenocarcinoma. A malignant tumor which has a nipple-like microscopic pattern; usually found in the bladder or ovary.

Polycythemia vera. A disease marked by the persistent increase of the red blood corpuscles.

Radioactive isotope. A chemical element which has been treated atomically to give off chemically active rays; used for diagnosis or used in lieu of X-ray treatment.

Sarcoma. A highly malignant tumor of connective tissue cells.

Short-circuiting surgery. Joining two parts of intestine above and below an obstruction.

Squamous cell carcinoma. A serious form of cancer which may occur in the lip, skin, mouth, lung, or cervix.

Stilbestrol. A synthetic sex hormone.

Testosterone. The male testicular hormone.

Tracheostomy. Operation to form an opening into the trachea through the neck.

Tracheotomy. The insertion of a tube through the operative opening into the trachea.

Undifferentiated tumor. A rapidly spreading and metastasizing malignant tumor.

References for Further Reading

I. BASIC SOCIAL WORK

Garrett, Annette. *Interviewing, Its Principles and Methods.* New York: Family Service Association of America, 1942.

Towle, Charlotte. *Common Human Needs.* New York: National Association of Social Workers, 1957.

U. S. Department of Health, Education, and Welfare, Social Security Administration, Bureau of Public Assistance. *More Than Bread,* by Helen C. Manning. Washington 25, D. C.: U. S. Government Printing Office, 1958.

U. S. Department of Health, Education, and Welfare, Social Security Administration, Bureau of Public Assistance. *The Role of the Caseworker,* by Helen B. Foster. Public Assistance Report No. 30. Washington 25, D. C.: U. S. Government Printing Office, 1956.

II. GENERAL MEDICAL

Dowling, Harry F., M.D., Sc.D., and Tom Jones, B.F.A. *That the Patient May Know.* Philadelphia and London: W. B. Saunders Company, 1959.

Facts on the Major Killing and Crippling Diseases in the United States Today. New York: National Health Education Committee, 1959.

Schifferes, Justus J., Ph.D. *Family Medical Encyclopedia*. New York: Permabooks, 1960.

Sproul, Edith E., M.D. *The Science Book of the Human Body*. Illustrated by Kathleen Elgin. New York: Pocket Books, Inc., 1959.

Swartz, Harry, M.D. *Intelligent Layman's Medical Dictionary*. New York: Frederick Ungar Publishing Co., 1955.

U. S. Department of Health, Education, and Welfare, Social Security Administration, Bureau of Old-Age and Survivors Insurance. *Description of Common Impairments*. Prepared by the Division of Disability Operations for the Use and Training of Administrative Staff. Washington: U. S. Government Printing Office, March, 1959.

III. SELECTED MEDICAL AND MEDICAL SOCIAL WORK

Arthritis and Related Disorders. Manual for Nurses, Physical Therapists and Medical Social Workers, 2d printing, issued by Medical and Scientific Committee, Arthritis and Rheumatism Foundation, New York.

Berlin, Irving, M.D. "A Review of Some Elements of Neurology: Parts I and II," *Social Casework,* 37 (November and December, 1956), 427–433, 493–500.

Cockerill, Eleanor. "The Social Worker Looks at Cancer." *In Readings in the Theory and Practice of Medical Social Work,* compiled by Dora Goldstine. Chicago: University of Chicago Press, 1954. Pp. 192–197.

"Community Approaches to the Problem of Tuberculosis," *Chronic Illness Newsletter,* 8 (December, 1957). Chicago: American Medical Association, 535 North Dearborn Street.

Elledge, Caroline H. *The Rehabilitation of the Patient*. Philadelphia, London, and Montreal: J. B. Lippincott Company.

Field, Minna. "Medical Social Work for the Aged." *In Read-*

ings in the Theory and Practice of Medical Social Work, compiled by Dora Goldstine. Chicago: University of Chicago Press, 1954. Pp. 264–273.

Field, Minna. *Patients Are People.* New York: Columbia University Press, 1958.

Gayford, Muriel. "Medical Social Work and Psychosomatic Medicine." *In Readings in the Theory and Practice of Medical Social Work,* compiled by Dora Goldstine. Chicago: University of Chicago Press, 1954. Pp. 140–152.

Glick, Selma J. *Vocational, Educational, and Recreational Needs of the Cerebral Palsied Adult.* Hunter College Chapter, International Council for Exceptional Children, April 1953. 1201–16th Street, N.W., Washington 6, D. C.

Ogg, Elizabeth. *When a Family Faces Cancer.* Public Affairs Pamphlet No. 286. New York: Public Affairs Committee, Inc. July, 1959.

Osteoarthritis, A Handbook for Patients. New York: The Arthritis and Rheumatism Foundation, 1958.

Primer for Paraplegics and Quadriplegics. Patient Publication No. 1, Institute of Physical Medicine and Rehabilitation. New York: University–Bellevue Medical Center, 1957.

Rice, Elizabeth P. "Co-operative Case Work." *In Readings in the Theory and Practice of Medical Social Work,* compiled by Dora Goldstine. Chicago: University of Chicago Press, 1954. Pp. 315–322.

Self-Help Devices for Rehabilitation. The National Foundation for Infantile Paralysis and New York University–Bellevue Medical Center. Dubuque, Iowa: William C. Brown Company, 1958.

Smith, Genevieve Waples, R.N., M.A. *Care of the Patient with a Stroke.* New York: Springer Publishing Co., Inc., 1959.

Strokes: A Guide for the Family. New York: American Heart Association, 1958.

Taylor, Martha. *Understanding Aphasia: A Guide for Family and Friends.* Patient Publication No. 2, Institute of Physical Medicine and Rehabilitation, New York: University–Bellevue Medical Center, 1958.

U. S. Department of Health, Education, and Welfare Office of Vocational Rehabilitation, *Psychological Aspects of Physical Disability*. Rehabilitation Service Series No. 210. Washington 25, D. C.: U. S. Government Printing Office, 194 pp.

U. S. Department of Health, Education, and Welfare Office of Vocational Rehabilitation, and Social Security Administration, Bureau of Public Assistance, *Working Together to Rehabilitate the Needy Disabled*. Prepared for State Public Assistance and Vocational Rehabilitation Programs, Washington 25, D. C.: U. S. Government Printing Office, 1955, 26 pp.

Bibliography

Chapter II: THE PSYCHOSOMATIC CONCEPT

Basowitz, Harold, M.D., and others. *Anxiety and Stress*. New York: McGraw-Hill Book Company, 1955.

Cannon, Walter, M.D. *Bodily Changes in Pain, Hunger, Fear and Rage*. New York: Appleton and Company, 1915.

Dunbar, Flanders, M.D. *Emotions and Bodily Changes*. 2d ed., New York: Columbia University Press, 1938.

Funkenstein, Daniel H., M.D., and others. *Mastery of Stress*. Cambridge: Harvard University Press, 1957.

Grollman, Arthur, M.D. "The Hypothalamus," *in Personality, Stress, and Tuberculosis*. Edited by Phenius J. Sparer, M.D. New York: International University Press, 1956, Chap. 2, pp. 16–27.

Selye, Hans, M.D. "Stress and Disease," *Geriatrics*, 10 (June, 1955), 253–261.

———. *The Stress of Life*. New York: McGraw-Hill Book Company, 1956.

Slaughter, Frank, M.D. *Medicine for Moderns*. New York: Messner Publishing Company, 1947.

Thewlis, Malford, M.D. "Stress and Longevity," *in The Care of the Aged*. St. Louis: C. V. Mosby Company, 1954, pp. 95–99.

Chapter III: RHEUMATOID ARTHRITIS

A Handbook on Rheumatoid Arthritis. New York: Arthritis and Rheumatism Foundation, 1956.

Arthritis. New York: Arthritis and Rheumatism Foundation.

Arthritis and Related Disorders (*Manual for Nurses, Physical Therapists and Medical Social Workers*). 2d printing, New York: Medical and Scientific Committee, Arthritis and Rheumatism Foundation.

Blair, Mary Grace, Ph.D., and Howard L. Holley, M.D. "Vitamin C and Rheumatoid Arthritis," *Journal of Chronic Diseases*, 4 (November, 1956), 549–551.

Blom, Gaston E., M.D., and Grace Nichols, M.S.S. "Emotional Factors in Children with Rheumatoid Arthritis," *American Journal of Orthopsychiatry, A Journal of Human Behavior*, 24 (July, 1954), 589–601.

Brown, Thomas McP., M.D., and others. "Rheumatoid Diseases and Gout," *in Long-Term Illness*. Edited by Michael G. Wohl, M.D. Philadelphia and London: W. B. Saunders Company, 1959, pp. 93–124.

Cecil, Russell L., M.D., Sc.D. *Diet and Your Arthritis and Other Facts About Arthritis*. Reprinted from *Look Magazine*. New York: Arthritis and Rheumatism Foundation. 1956.

Clark, William S., M.D., and others. "Rehabilitation of Patients with Rheumatoid Arthritis," *Journal of Chronic Diseases*, 5 (June, 1957), 712–722.

Cobb, Sidney, M.D. M.P.H. and others. "An Estimate of the Prevalance of Rheumatoid Arthritis" *Journal of Chronic Diseases*, 5 (June, 1957), 636–643.

Description of Arthritis and Nonarticular Rheumatism. Sacramento: California State Department of Social Welfare, February, 1958.

Freyberg, R. H., M.D. "The Use of Hormones in Rheumatic Disorders," *Journal of Chronic Diseases,* 2 (November, 1955), 559–582.

King, Stanley H., Ph.D. "Psychological Factors Associated with Rheumatoid Arthritis: An Evaluation of the Literature," *Journal of Chronic Diseases,* 2 (September, 1955), 287–302.

Kuzell, William C., M.D., and others. "Some Observations on 520 County Patients," *Journal of Chronic Diseases,* 2 (December, 1955), 645–669.

Lewin, Philip, M.D. *Arthritis and the Rheumatic Diseases.* New York: McGraw-Hill Book Company, 1951.

Lowman, Edward W., M.D. "Rehabilitation of the Patient with Chronic Rheumatoid Arthritis: A Two-Year Study," *Journal of Chronic Diseases,* 1 (June, 1955), 628–637.

———. "Self-Help Devices for the Arthritic." *Rehabilitation Monograph VI.* New York University–Bellevue Medical Center, Institute of Physical Medicine and Rehabilitation.

Manheimer, Robert H., M.D., and Martin Acker, B.S. "Back to Work, Program for Physically Handicapped Arthritics," *Journal of Chronic Diseases,* 5 (June, 1957), 770–778.

Osteoarthritis, A Handbook for Patients. New York: Arthritis and Rheumatism Foundation, 1958, pp. 1–20.

Ragan, Charles, M.D. "The Present-Day Management of Arthritis," *Journal of Chronic Diseases,* 1 (March, 1955), 253–265.

Schless, Bessie G. "Social Casework Services to the Arthritic Patient," *The Family* (*Journal of Social Casework*), 25 (January, 1945), 331–336.

Stop Arthritis: Symptoms and Treatment. San Francisco: Arthritis and Rheumatism Foundation, Northern California Chapter.

Chapter IV: DIABETES MELLITUS

Cecil, Russell L., M.D., ScD., and Robert F. Loeb, M.D., eds. "Diabetes Mellitus," *in Textbook of Medicine.* Philadelphia and London: W. B. Saunders Company, 1955, pp. 658–681.

Danowski, T. S., M.D. *Diabetes as a Way of Life*. New York: Coward-McCann, 1957.

Ditzel, Jørn, M.D., and Priscilla White, M.D. "Central Retinal Vein Occlusion in Juvenile Diabetes," *Journal of Chronic Diseases*, 3 (March, 1956), 253–261.

Dobson, Harold L., M.D., and others. "Socioeconomic Status and Diabetes Mellitus," *Journal of Chronic Diseases*, 7 (May, 1958), 415–421.

Duncan, Garfield, M.D. *A Modern Pilgrim's Progress for Diabetes*. Philadelphia and London: W. B. Saunders Company, 1956.

Hinkle, Lawrence E., Jr., M.D., and Stewart Wolf, M.D. "Importance of Life Stress in Course and Management of Diabetes Mellitus," *Journal of the American Medical Association*, Vol. 48, Pt. 1. January–February, 1952, pp. 513–520.

Iskrant, Albert P., M.A., and Arnold B. Kurlander, M.D. "Diabetes Mellitus Mortality in the Continental United States 1950," *Journal of Chronic Diseases*, 1 (April, 1955), 368–380.

LeCompte, Philip M., M.D. "Vascular Lesions in Diabetes Mellitus," *Journal of Chronic Diseases*, 2 (August, 1955), 178–215.

Mitchell, Roger S., M.D. "Present Day Management of Tuberculosis," *Journal of Chronic Diseases*, 4 (December, 1956), 627.

O'Donovan, C. J., M.D. "New Orally Effective Adjuvants in the Management of Diabetes Mellitus," *Journal of Chronic Diseases*, 4 (December, 1956), 627.

Root, Howard F., M.D., FACP, Sc.D. "Treatment of Diabetic Coma," *Journal of Chronic Diseases*, 2 (August, 1955), 121–135.

Root, Howard F., M.D., and Priscilla White, M.D. "Diabetes Mellitus-Handbook for Physicians," *Journal of Chronic Diseases*, 5 (May, 1957), 606.

U. S. Department of Health, Education, and Welfare. *Taking*

Care of Diabetes. Public Health Service Publication No. 567. Washington, 1957.

Wilkerson, Hugh L. C., M.D. and others. "Screening for Diabetes," *Journal of Chronic Diseases,* 2 (October, 1955), 464.

Zeman, Frederic D., M.D. "Genetic Factors in the Diseases of Later Life," *Journal of Chronic Diseases,* 2 (July, 1955), 14.

Chapter V:TUBERCULOSIS

Alcoholic Rehabilitation Commission. Final Report. Berkeley, California, September 4, 1957.

"The Big Headache," *The California State Employee,* 30 (February, 1959).

Block, Marvin A., M.D. "Alcoholism Is a Disease." Reprinted from *Today's Health,* American Medical Association, 1956.

Blomquist, Edward T., M.D. "The Nonhospitalized Tuberculosis Patient." Reprinted from *American Journal of Public Health,* 46 (February, 1956).

Boock, James J. (Chief GA-AND Division, Sacramento County Department of Public Welfare). Unpublished material.

Daniel, Beryl, and Gordon V. Hromadka. *The Lost Patient* (Investigation into Problems of Recalcitrancy). San Francisco: California Tuberculosis and Health Association, 1957.

Digest of Findings of PHS Study of Nonhospitalized Patients and PHS Recommendations for Improvement in TB Control Programs. New York: National Tuberculosis Association, 1956.

"Dx: Tuberculosis—Rx: Total Rehabilitation," *Rehabilitation Events,* 3 (June, 1957), National Tuberculosis Association.

Dx Tuberculosis—Rx: Total Rehabilitation (The Technical Report of the Study of the Rehabilitation Needs of the Tuberculous in California). San Francisco: Social Research Division, California Tuberculosis and Health Association, 1955–1956.

Golder, Grace, R.N. "Some Aspects of the Relationship of

Alcoholism and Tuberculosis." Reprinted from *Connecticut Review on Alcoholism,* 3 (January, 1952).

"Homemaker Service A New Aid to Tuberculosis Patients," *Rehabilitation Events,* 3 (September, 1957), National Tuberculosis Association.

Hummel, Joan, Research Associate. *The Alcoholic Tuberculous Patient* (A Supplementary to the Study of the Rehabilitation Needs of the Tuberculous in California). San Francisco: California Tuberculosis and Health Association, 1956.

"Interest is Increasing in Analyzing Characteristics of Nonrehabilitated Patients," *Rehabilitation Events,* 2 (September, 1956), National Tuberculosis Association.

"Is Social Work Important in Tuberculosis Clinic Programs?" *Rehabilitation Events,* 1, (November, 1955), National Tuberculosis Association.

Loos, Gertrude. "The Challenge of the Future," *Rehabilitation Events,* National Tuberculosis Association.

————. Speech which might be given by a paid executive at an annual meeting of a tuberculosis association, December 6, 1956.

McCarthy, Raymond G., ed. *Drinking and Intoxication.* Publications Division, Yale Center of Alcohol Studies, New Haven, Connecticut. Glencoe, Illinois: The Free Press, 1959.

Morse, Dan, M.D. "Alcohol and Tuberculosis." Reprinted from the NTA Bulletin (November, 1956).

Problems of the Recalcitrant Tuberculosis Patient in California. San Francisco: Social Research Division, California Tuberculosis and Health Association, 1956–1957.

"Public Assistance Has a Major Role in Tuberculosis Control," *Rehabilitation Events,* 2 (May, 1956), National Tuberculosis Association.

"Rehabilitation of the Tuberculosis Aging—The Stage is Set." *Rehabilitation Events,* 3 (March, 1957), National Tuberculosis Association.

Summary Report of the Study of the Rehabilitation Needs of the Tuberculosus in California. California Tuberculosis and Health Association, May 3, 1954—June 30, 1956.

"Target: Community Action." *Rehabilitation Events,* 3 (December, 1957), National Tuberculosis Association.

Trends in Tuberculosis. New York: National Tuberculosis Association, 1958.

U. S. Department of Health, Education, and Welfare, Division of Special Service Tuberculosis Program. *Tuberculosis Chart Series 1957,* Public Health Service Publication No. 534. Washington, 1957.

"Volunteers in Action. *"Rehabilitation Events,* 4 (March, 1958), National Tuberculosis Association.

"What Is Your Community Doing about Alcoholic Tuberculosis Patients?" *Rehabilitation Events,* 2 (December, 1956), National Tuberculosis Association.

Chapter VI: THE PULMONARY CRIPPLE

Cecil, Russell L., M.D., Sc.D., and Robert F. Loeb, M.D., eds. "Asthma," pp. 474–482, "Chronic Emphysema," pp. 1031–1036, in *Textbook of Medicine.* Philadelphia and London: W. B. Saunders Company, 1955.

Hanson-Pruss, O. C., and John D. Charlton. "Emphysema in the Aged," *American Geriatrics Journal,* 2 (1954), 153–170.

Hinshaw, Corwin H., and Henry L. Garland. "Bronchial Asthma and Related Conditions," pp. 228–244, "Pulmonary Emphysema," pp. 245–266, in *Diseases of the Chest.* Philadelphia and London: W. B. Saunders Company, 1956.

Miller, R. Drew. "Management of Diffuse Obstructive Pulmonary Emphysema," *American Geriatrics Society Journal,* 2 (1954), 502–508.

Rappaport, Israel, and Edgar Mayer. "Emphysema and the Senile Lung," *American Geriatrics Society Journal,* 2 (1954), 581–591.

Snyder, James. "Relation of Disability to Hypoxemia and Congestive Failure in Pulmonary Emphysema," *U. S. Armed Forces Medical Journal,* 8 (1957), 1577–1589.

Trimble, Harold G., and James Kieran. "Pulmonary Emphysema Treated by Intermittent Positive Pressure Breathing," *American Geriatrics Society Journal,* 2 (1954), 102–107.

Chapter VII: PROGRESSIVE DISEASES OF THE
NERVOUS SYSTEM

Berlin, Irving, M.D. "A Review of Some Elements of Neurol-
ogy: Parts I and II," *Social Casework,* 37 (November and
December, 1956), 427–433, 493–500.
Cecil, Russell L., M.D., Sc.D., and Robert F. Loeb, M.D., eds.
Textbook of Medicine. Philadelphia and London: W. B.
Saunders Company, 1951, pp. 1406–1414; 1514–1520;
1530–1535; 1536–1560; 1582–1584.
Critchley, MacDonald, M.D. "Neurological Changes in the
Aged," *Journal of Chronic Diseases,* 3 (May, 1956), 459–
476.
"Out of the Shadows." Public Affairs Pamphlet No. 271, New
York.
Schumacher, George A., M.D. "Multiple Sclerosis," *Journal of
Chronic Diseases,* 8 (October, 1958), 464–484.
Schwabe, Robert, M.D., and Gilbert England, M.D. "Parkin-
son's Disease," *Journal of Chronic Diseases,* 8 (October,
1958), 488–509.
Schwarz, Gabriel A., M.D., and Geraldine King, M.D. "Neuro-
muscular Diseases of Later Maturity: Part I," *Geriatrics,* 10
(May, 1955), 197–206.
U. S. Department of Health, Education, and Welfare. *Multiple
Sclerosis: Hope Through Research.* Public Health Series Pub-
lication No. 621, Health Information Series No. 92, Washington.

Chapter VIII: EPILEPSY

Bradley, Charles, M.D. "Treatment of a Convulsive Child in a
Children's Psychiatric Hospital." Reprinted from *The Ner-
vous Child,* 6 (1947). National Epilepsy League.
Cecil, Russell L., M.D., Sc.D., and Robert F. Loeb, M.D., eds.
Textbook of Medicine. 8th ed., Philadelphia and London:
W. B. Saunders Company, 1951, pp. 1486–1495.

Cummins, Jean. "The Family as a Factor in the Epileptic's Social Adjustment," *Journal of Social Casework* (November, 1949), 384–387.

Davidson, Elabel McL., and Joan C. Thomas. "A Social Study of Epileptic Patients," *Journal of Social Casework* (November, 1949), 380–383.

Education for All American Children. Jointly published by International Council on Exceptional Children and The National Epilepsy League.

Gibbs, Frederic A., M.D. "A Modern View of Epilepsy." (An address made before the 26th Annual Conference of the International Council for Exceptional Children at Des Moines, Iowa, April 26, 1958), National Epilepsy League.

Hammill, James F., M.D. "Epilepsy," *Journal of Chronic Diseases,* 8 (October, 1958), 448–463.

Lennox, William G., M.D. "The Epileptic Patient and the Nurse," *American Journal of Nursing,* 46 (April, 1946).

———. "Marriage and Children for Epileptics," *Human Fertility,* 10 (December, 1945). National Epilepsy League.

Lennox, William G., M.D., and Stanley Cobb, M.D. *The Employment of Epileptics—Facts, Not Superstitions,* National Epilepsy League.

Merritt, Houston H., M.D. "Treatment of Epilepsy," *Cincinnati Journal of Medicine,* 1946. National Epilepsy League.

Miers, Earl Schenck. *Why Did This Have to Happen: An Open Letter to Parents.* Parent Series No. 1, National Society for Crippled Children and Adults, Inc., 1957.

Pinanski, Joan. *Social Service and Seizures: Information about Epilepsy for the Social Worker.* National Epilepsy League, February 21, 1946.

Symposium on the Convulsive Disorders. The Medical Clinics of North America. Philadelphia and London: W. B. Saunders Company, 1958.

   Conn, Howard F., M.D. "Extracerebral Causes of Seizures," pp. 337–344.

   Crawley, James W., M.D. "The Overall Management of the Adult Epileptic," pp. 317–326.

Fabing, Howard D., M.D. "Epilepsy and the Law," pp. 361–374.

Harvald, B., M.D. "Hereditary Factors in Epilepsy," pp. 345–348.

Kellaway, Peter, A.M., Ph.D., and Ralph Druckman, M.D. "Idiopathic Epilepsy: Criteria for Diagnosis," pp. 375–378.

Richardson, Edward P., Jr., M.D. "Late Life Epilepsy," pp. 349–360.

Ward, Arthur A., Jr. "The Surgical Treatment of Epilepsy," pp. 327–336.

Yahraes, Herbert, *Epilepsy: The Ghost Is out of the Closet.* Public Affairs Pamphlet, No. 98, December, 1944.

Chapter IX: CEREBRAL PALSY

Abbott, Marguerite. *Cerebral Palsy—Its Scope and Management.* Public Affairs Pamphlet No. 158A, February, 1956.

Bobath, Karel, M.D., and Mrs. *Physical Therapy Demonstration and Discussion.* The Work Conference on the Rehabilitation Process, Sheltered Workshops and Special Techniques in Physical Therapy, San Francisco State College, July, 1958, pp. 32–54.

Cardwell, Viola E. *Cerebral Palsy: Advances in Understanding and Care.* Association for the Aid of Crippled Children, 1956.

Clark, Randolph Lee, Jr., B.S., M.D., M.Sc., and Russell W. Cumley, B.A., M.A., Ph.D., eds., "Cerebral Palsy," in *Family Health Encyclopedia.* New York: Little and Ives, 1956, Vol. 3, pp. 616–622.

Cruickshank, William M., Ph.D., and George M. Raus, M.D. *Cerebral Palsy: Its Individual and Community Problems.* Syracuse: Syracuse University Press, 1955.

Deaver, George G., M.D. "Cerebral Palsy: Methods of Evaluation and Treatment," *Rehabilitation Monograph IX,* New York: University–Bellevue Medical Center, Institute of Physical Medicine and Rehabilitation, 1955.

Glick, Selma J. *Vocational, Educational, and Recreational Needs of the Cerebral Palsied Adult.* New York: Hunter College Chapter, International Council for Exceptional Children, April, 1953.

Miers, Earl Schenck. *Why Did This Have to Happen: An Open Letter to Parents.* Parent Series No. 1, The National Society for Crippled Children and Adults, 1957.

Phelps, Winthrop M., M.D. "Cerebral Palsy," in *Long-term Illness.* Edited by Michael G. Wohl, M.D., Philadelphia and London: W. B. Saunders Company, 1959, pp. 462–469.

Schlesigner, Edward R., M.D., and others. "Survivorship in Cerebral Palsy," *American Journal of Public Health,* 49 (March, 1959), 343–348.

Spencer, Helen, RPT. *A Glossary of Scientific Terms in the Field of Cerebral Palsy.* Department of Physical Medicine and Rehabilitation, College of Physicians and Surgeons, New York: Columbia University, March, 1956.

Chapter X: PARAPLEGIA AND QUADRIPLEGIA

Bennett, Robert L., M.D. "Management of the Patient with Severe Chronic Poliomyelitis," in *Long-Term Illness.* Edited by Michael G. Wohl, M.D. Philadelphia and London: W. B. Saunders Company, 1959, pp. 437–444.

Bors, Ernest, M.D. "Spinal Cord Injury," in *Long-Term Illness.* Edited by Michael G. Wohl, M.D. Philadelphia and London: W. B. Saunders Company, 1959, pp. 469–479.

Grant, Alice A., "Medical Social Work in an Epidemic of Polio," *Journal of Pediatrics,* 24 (June, 1944), 691–723.

Homberger, Freddy, M.D. *The Medical Care of the Aged and Chronically Ill.* Boston: Little, Brown and Company, 1955, pp. 158–178.

Lassen, H. C. A., M.D. "Management of Respiratory and Bulbar Paralysis in Poliomyelitis," in *Poliomyelitis.* Geneva: World Health Organization, 1955, pp. 157–211.

Primer for Paraplegics and Quadriplegics. Patient Publication No. 1, The Institute of Physical Medicine and Rehabilitation,

New York: University–Bellevue Medical Center, 1957.

Rosenblatt, Aaron, and Vincent W. Trovato. "Evaluating a Medical Symptom with Paraplegics," *Social Casework,* XLI (March, 1960), 128–134.

U. S. Department of Health, Education, and Welfare, Children's Bureau, Social Security Administration, *Infantile Paralysis,* prepared by American Orthopedic Association, Washington, 1946.

Wechsler, Israel S., M.D. *A Textbook of Clinical Neurology.* 8th ed., Illustrated, Philadelphia and London: W. B. Saunders Company, 1958, pp. 103–108.

Chapter XI: CARDIOVASCULAR DISEASE AND DISEASES OF THE OUTLYING VESSELS

Benedict, Ruth B., M.D. "Onset and Early Course of Essential Hypertension," *Journal of Chronic Diseases,* 4 (September, 1956), 221–230.

Cecil, Russell L., M.D., Sc.D., and Robert F. Loeb, M.D., eds., "Diseases of the Cardiovascular System," in *Textbook of Medicine.* 9th ed., Philadelphia and London: W. B. Saunders Company, 1955, pp. 1230–1258; 1291–1303; 1319–1337; 1376–1403.

Clark, Randolph Lee, Jr., B.S., M.D., M.Sc., and Russell W. Cumley, B.A., M.A., Ph.D., eds. *Family Health Encyclopedia.* 2d printing. New York: J. J. Little and Ives Publishing Co., Inc., 1956, Vol. 2, 327–335; Vol. 2, 355–364; Vol. 3, 695–712; Vol. 6, 1432–1441.

Haselkorn, Florence, and Leopold Bellak, M.D. "A Multiple Service Approach to Cardiac Patients," *Social Casework,* 21 (July, 1950), 292–298.

Hilleboe, Herman E., M.D. "Some Epidemiologic Aspects of Coronary Artery Disease," *Journal of Chronic Diseases,* 6 (September, 1957), 210–228.

Levy, Robert L., M.D. "Current Views on Certain Aspects of

Management in Cardiac Infarction," *Journal of Chronic Diseases,* 4 (October, 1956), 332–339.

"The Prevention of Rheumatic Fever," *Public Health Reports,* Vol. 68, No. 1 (January, 1953).

Smith, Mary Alice, M.D. "A Community Program for the Prevention of Rheumatic Fever Recurrence," *Public Health Reports,* Vol. 68, No. 1 (January, 1953), 16–19.

Stewart, William H., and Philip E. Enterline. "Ecology and Coronary Heart Disease," *Journal of Chronic Diseases,* 6 (July, 1957), 86–89.

Chapter XII: CEREBRAL VASCULAR DISEASE

Alvarez, Walter C., M.D., F.A.C.P. "The Abdominal Symptoms of Little Strokes," *Geriatrics,* 12 (March, 1957).

————. "Cerebral Arteriosclerosis with Small Commonly Unrecognized Apoplexies," *Geriatrics,* 1 (May-June, 1946), 189–216.

————. "Management of Small Strokes," *Geriatrics,* 12 (July, 1957), 421–425.

Baker, Lenox D., M.D. "Neuromuscular Problems in Hemiplegic and Paraplegic Patients," *Geriatrics* (October, 1956), 434–439.

Bortz, Edward L., M.D. "Mastering Long-Term Illness," *Geriatrics,* 11 (October, 1956), 447–452.

Cecil, Russell L., M.D., Sc.D., and Robert F. Loeb, M.D., eds. "Atherosclerosis," pp. 697–701; "Senile Heart Diseases," pp. 1317–1318; "Aphasia," pp. 1499–1503; "Hemiplegia," pp. 1503–1508; "Diffuse and Focal Diseases of the Brain," pp. 1585–1600. *In Textbook of Medicine.* 9th ed., Philadelphia and London: W. B. Saunders Company, 1955.

Cerebral Vascular Disease and Strokes—*Diseases of the Blood Vessels of the Brain (Cerebral Vascular Disease).* Prepared by the Heart Information Center, National Heart Institute, Washington: Government Printing Office, 1957, p. 5.

Covalt, Donald A., M.D. "After Care of the Hemiplegic," Reprinted from *GP,* II (September, 1950).

————. "Early Management of a Patient with a Stroke," Reprinted from *Medical Times* 86, (April, 1958).

Cowdry, E. V., M.D. ed. *The Care of the Geriatric Patient.* St. Louis: C. V. Mosby Co., 1958.

Denken, Harold, M.D. "Physical Treatment of the Hemiplegic Patient in General Practice," *Journal of the American Medical Association,* 139 (April 30, 1949), 1255–1259.

Ehrentheil, Otto F. "Differential Diagnosis of Organic Dementias and Affective Disorders in the Aged," *Geriatrics,* 12 (July, 1957), 426–432.

Fazekas, Joseph F., M.D., and others. "Evaluation of Current Therapy in Cerebral Vascular Disease," *Journal of Chronic Diseases,* 2 (November, 1955), 508–518.

Feldman, Louis, M.D. "A Positive Approach to Management of Cerebro-Vascular Accident," *Geriatrics,* 6 (July-August, 1951), 214–220.

Lee, Philip R., M.D., and others. "An Evaluation of Rehabilitation of Patients with Hemiparesis or Hemiplegia Due to Cerebral Vascular Disease." *Rehabilitation Monograph XV,* The Institute of Physical Medicine and Rehabilitation, New York: University–Bellevue Medical Center, 1958.

Lewis, Howard P., M.D., ed. "Genetic Factors in Cardiovascular Diseases: II. Disorders of Primarily Genetic Etiology," *Modern Concepts of Cardiovascular Disease,* Vol. XXVIII, No. 8 (August, 1959), New York: American Heart Association.

————. "Strokes—Diagnosis and Modern Treatment: II. Treatment," *Modern Concepts of Cardiovascular Disease,* Vol. XXVIII, No. 5 (May, 1959), New York: American Heart Association.

Linden, Maurice E., M.D. "Cultural and Socio-psychological Considerations in Work with the Aged," *Social Casework,* XL (November, 1959).

Macrae, Donald, M.D., and Robert B. Aird, M.D. "Diseases of the Nervous System," *in Long-Term Illness.* Edited by

Michael G. Wohl, M.D. Philadelphia and London: W. B. Saunders Company, 1959, pp. 403–412.

Neugartey, Bernice, and David Garron. "Attitudes of Middle-Aged Person toward Growing Older," *Geriatrics,* 14 (January, 1959).

Peszczynski, Mieczyslaw, M.D. "Prevention of Falls in the Hemiplegic Patient," *Geriatrics,* 11 (July, 1956), 306–311.

"Preventive Geriatrics," *Journal of Michigan State Medical Society,* Vol. 56, No. 5 (May, 1957).

Stieglitz, Edward J., M.D. "Nutrition Problems of Geriatric Medicine," *Journal of the American Medical Association,* 142 (January-April, 1950).

Strokes: A Guide for the Family, New York: American Heart Association, 1958.

Taylor, Martha. *Understanding Aphasia: A Guide for Family and Friends,* Patient Publication No. 2, Institute of Physical Medicine and Rehabilitation, New York: University–Bellevue Medical Center, 1958.

U. S. Department of Health, Education, and Welfare, Public Health Services. *The Older Person in the Home,* Public Health Services Publication No. 342, Washington: Government Printing Office, 1957.

————. *Strike Back at Stroke,* Public Health Services Publication No. 596, Washington: Government Printing Office, 1958.

Warren, Marjory, M.D. "Queries and Therapeutic Notes: Treatment of Hemiplegia of an Old Person in a Private Home," *Geriatrics,* 12 (April, 1957).

Weil, Julius, Ph.D. "Special Services for the Senile in a Home for the Aged," *Geriatrics,* 9 (September, 1954), 443–445.

"What Are the Facts About Arteriosclerosis Our Number One Killer?" *Facts on the Major Killing and Crippling Diseases in the United States Today,* Compiled by the National Health Education Committee, Inc. New York, 1959 ed., pp. 1–17.

Young, Wei, B.S. and others. "The Interrelationship between Cerebral and Coronary Atherosclerosis," *Geriatrics,* 11 (September, 1956), 413–418.

Chapter XIII: CANCER

Abrams, Ruth D. "Social Casework with Cancer Patients," *Social Casework,* 32 (December, 1951), 425–432.

Aust, J. B., M.D., and Claude R. Hitchcock, M.D. "Scientific Exhibit: Minnesota Cancer Detection Research Center, a Six-Year Report," *Geriatrics,* 10 (March, 1955), 105–110.

Berman, Edgar F., M.D. "Carcinoma of the Esophagus: A Geriatric Problem," *Geriatrics,* 9 (November, 1954), 520–523.

Bibliography on Cancer for Nurses. New York: American Cancer Society, Medical Library, Medical and Scientific Department.

Cancer and the Nursing Profession, New York: American Cancer Society, 1957.

A Cancer Source Book for Nurses, New York: American Cancer Society, 1950.

Cecil, Russell L., M.D., Sc.D., and Robert F. Loeb, M.D., eds. *Textbook of Medicine.* 8th ed., Philadelphia and London: W. B. Saunders Company, 1951, pp. 906–909, 1042–1045, 1214–1223.

Clark, Randolph Lee, Jr., B.S., M.D., M.Sc., and Russell W. Cumley, B.A., M.A., Ph.D., eds. *Family Health Encyclopedia.* 2d printing. New York: J. J. Little and Ives Publishing Co., Inc., 1956, Vol. 2, pp. 342–349.

Conley, John J., M.D. "Significance of Cancer of the Head and Neck in the Aged," *Geriatrics,* 13 (April, 1958), 197–201.

Costello, Cyril, M.D. "Earlier Diagnosis in Cancer of the Colon," *Geriatrics,* 9 (March, 1954), 116–120.

Crile, George, Jr., M.D. "Adenoma and Carcinoma of the Thyroid," *Geriatrics,* 9 (April, 1954), 146–148.

Davidoff, Reuben B., M.D. "Occult Carcinoma of the Breast," *Geriatrics,* 9 (March, 1954), 128–129.

Glassman, William S., M.D., and Paul W. Johnston, M.D. "Palliative Surgery in Carcinoma of the Pancreas," *Geriatrics,* 10 (October, 1955), 456–458.

Hahn, George A., M.D. "Radioisotopes in the Treatment of Pelvic Cancer," *Geriatrics,* 11 (March, 1956), 113–118.

Homburger, Freddy, M.D. "The Care of Patients with Advanced Cancer" (Symposium: Care of the Elderly Cancer Patient), *Geriatrics,* 11 (September, 1956), 372–385.

Johnson, Dallas. *Facing the Facts About Cancer,* Public Affairs Pamphlet No. 38, (Revised), 1956, American Cancer Society and the National Cancer Institute of the U.S. Public Health Service.

Joost, A. M. Meerloo, M.D. "Psychologic Implications of Cancer," *Geriatrics,* 9 (April, 1954), 154–156.

Murray, Foster, M.D. "Diagnosis and Treatment of Lung Cancer," *Geriatrics,* 10 (March, 1955), 118–122.

Narrowing the Search, New York City Cancer Committee of American Cancer Society.

Nelson, H. M. (University of Michigan M. Bull. 23: 419–425, 1957), "The Present Status of Exfoliative Cytology in the Control of Uterine Cancer," Digest of Current Literature, *Geriatrics,* 13 (April, 1958), 82a.

Newell, R. R., M.D. "What Should We Tell the Patient," *Journal of Chronic Diseases,* 7 (January, 1958), 52–57.

Scheele, Leonard A., M.D., and Herman E. Hilleboe, M.D. *Cancer Nursing—A Manual for Public Health Nurses,* Revised 1955, Joint project of National Cancer Institute, Public Health Service, Department of Health, Education, and Welfare, and the New York State Department of Health.

TeLinde, Richard W. "Carcinoma of the Corpus Uteri," *in Operative Gynecology,* 2d ed., pp. 455–465.

———. "Choice of Treatment" (Subsection of chapter on "Cancer of the Cervix Uteri"), *in Operative Gynecology,* 2d ed., pp. 401–423.

U. S. Department of Health, Education, and Welfare, Public Health Service, *Reading on Cancer—An Annotated Bibliography,* Public Health Bibliography Series No. 14, 1955, Prepared by Office of Information and Publication, National Cancer Institute.

Youth Looks at Cancer—An Information Text for College Preparatory School and High School Students. American Cancer Society, Inc., The Westchester Cancer Committee, 18th ed., 1956.

Index